To Pete

Keep Your Voice
Strong &
Your
Vision
Clear!

Best Wishes,

Michael

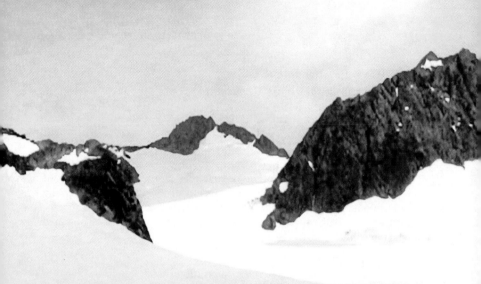

VOICES FROM THE EDGE

Life Lessons from the Cancer Community

MICHAEL HAYES SAMUELSON

LONGSTREET PRESS

ATLANTA

VOICES FROM THE EDGE
Life Lessons from the Cancer Community
Michael H. Samuelson

Longstreet Press
2140 Newmarket Parkway, Suite 122
Marietta, Georgia 30067
800-927-1488 or 770-980-1488 voice, 770-859-9894 fax

Library of Congress catalog card number: 00-108698

ISBN: 1-56352-644-1 hardcover

The author may be contacted at the following address:

Samuelson & Associates
3055 Plymouth Road, Suite 202
Ann Arbor, MI 48105
734-747-9579, fax 734-429-3346
msamuelson2@msn.com

CREDITS
Developmental Editing: **Jeff Morris**
Copyediting: **Deborah Costenbader**
Proofreading: **Deborah Costenbader**
Text Design/Production: **Jeff Morris**
Photography: **Derek and Michael Samuelson**
Jacket Design: **Burtch Hunter, Jeff Morris**

First printing: October 2000

This book is dedicated to the men, women, and children of the worldwide cancer community.

CONTENTS

Acknowledgments

. . . WHERE TO BEGIN?

The individuals whose voices constitute the heart of this book are very special people. I am grateful beyond expression for the chance to know them and for the opportunity to bring their stories to print. More than their words, they shared their tears, laughter, anger, frustrations, hopes, and dreams. They allowed themselves to once again become vulnerable so that we might learn from their travels. Thank you, Tim, Lillie, Lou, Fern, Matthew, Ricky, Doug, Paula, and Hank. Thanks also to Max, Jack, Laurette, and the dozens of other community members I have met during my short time in our town.

A huge thank you to my brother David Samuelson, a talented writer, editor, and trusted friend who continually pointed me in the right direction, kept me on task, and taught me more than he'll ever know he did. I may be in my fifties, but he is still my big brother, and it's comforting to know he's always in my corner.

The "Yes We Can!" award goes to Scott Bard and his staff at Longstreet Press. High-quality production in the sweep of a stopwatch. Remarkable efficiency!

Thanks also to these people:

Jeff Morris, who put it all together while dealing with both impossible deadlines and an author who kept making last-minute (last-second) changes. Quite simply, this book never would have made it to press on time without Jeff's dedication and talent.

Suzanne Mahler, Jane Spinner, Elena Weisman, Andrew Samuelson, Jessica Ludy, Jennifer Kupz, John Hoben, and many others who read parts of the manuscript and offered excellent feedback.

Carmen Ludy, who stood by me and my family in more ways than this book has pages.

Connie Doyle and Alan Dempsky, who have been at my side for close to thirty years.

My associate, Karen Revill, who keeps me organized, makes my excuses, and reminds me what time zone I'm in.

Tim Murnane, for his encouragement to start this project, his great baseball playing at Tiger Stadium, and our friendship breaks at Zola's Cafe.

Rod Byrne, whose compassion and sharing of information led directly to the early detection that saved my life, and who was there at the hospital when they wheeled me in and wheeled me out.

My mother-in-law, Florence Muhmey, who was by my side at the hospital; my brother Paul, his wife, Joan, and their family; and my sister-in-law, Anne Farrell, and her family.

A very special twenty-two-year thank you to Tom Connellan, my mentor, friend, guide, cheerleader, confessor, and inspiration. He is always, always there for me whenever I reach out for help and, more important, when I don't think I need any.

Finally, and most important, the people who make sense out of my life: Hillary, my wife, dearest friend, staunchest supporter, and most honest critic; and my children, Brent, Derek, and Logan. We laugh, we cry, we whisper, and sometimes (not very often) we raise our voices — but most of all, we like and we love.

"HOW COULD YOU CHOOSE SUCH A DEPRESSING FIELD AS ONCOLOGY?"
Oncologists get asked this question again and again. My short
answer is that cancer care is one of the most inspiring areas of medicine, and rarely depressing. This statement is usually met with a quiz-
zical look. My shorter answer is the chance to meet cancer's heroes
and their remarkable response to adversity. This answer still seems
to cause puzzlement. Now, with the publication of Michael
Samuelson's *Voices from the Edge,* I have a better and more complete
answer to the question.

The healing of life through serious illness is an unfamiliar theme
in the Western world and its medicine. We see no point to illness. It
is futile suffering to no end, and we seek the cure, not its meaning.
When we talk of healing, we mean healing of illness, not healing
through illness. However, as natural as our own view seems to us, it is
not the way other cultures have traditionally looked upon illness.

So alien to modern medicine is the notion of healing through
illness that I can recall only one mention in medical training of illness having a positive effect. We were learning about bed-wetters and
the fact that the most refractory cases of bed-wetting resolve themselves after a serious illness. Somehow, battling illness brings a child
naturally to a higher level of maturity. The instructor argued, a bit
flippantly, that the best prescription for bed-wetting is a viral illness.

Recently the world witnessed dramatic and overwhelming evidence of maturity through illness. During the 2000 Tour de France,
a day of wind, rain, and temperatures in the thirties became for the
world's top bike racers a dark night of the soul — all but one. Lance
Armstrong did his warm-ups with gusto. It was a day that separated
the Man from the men — a breakaway day. Lance had already faced
death (or to put it more bluntly, annihilation) and had overcome

bouts of impossible misery during his therapy. On his scale of adversity, this did not meet the mark of a miserable day. The question we might ask is, Did Lance Armstrong win in spite of cancer, or because of cancer?

In this collection, we do not meet famous survivors accomplishing the impossible. This is the strength of the manuscript, rather than a weakness. If transformation is reserved to an outstanding few, of what use is it to ordinary folk? Even Bernie Segal, in *Love, Medicine, and Miracles*, implied that only a subgroup of his patients had the take-charge, responsible attitude of the winner. I have trouble with this winners-and-losers categorization. In my practice, I believe that each patient displays the heroic response to whatever degree possible, and it is destructive to disparage those who overcome a little, rather than overcome completely. Michael has populated a book with ordinary people, as did Thornton Wilder his wonderful play *Our Town* — but look closely. The town Michael's people reside in is consciousness, courage, appreciation, humor, and grace. It is a town of humans carried beyond themselves to another level of being.

This book is an intimate portrait of Michael's townspeople — the cancer community. I marvel and wonder at the degree of intimacy. Because Michael is a fellow patient, he earned the trust that allowed these subjects to share themselves completely. There may be another reason for this disclosure as well. One mark of the cancer experience might be easy access to the deeper self. Cancer patients have, after all, been digging deep into themselves for the strength to endure and have found both great strengths and great weaknesses. In other words, they know themselves and are more comfortable with themselves than those less tested. They freely reveal private thoughts that those with less insight might be embarrassed by.

The portraits are fair and diverse. There are those who turn to their spouses and loving families for support, but there are just as many stories of single parents raising families alone who must look elsewhere. Often, patients look to people they met decades before. Cancer not only tests our life at the point of diagnosis, it tests our whole life. We may invoke pithy single lines of advice heard first in childhood but raised now as inspiring battle cries. We may recall a childhood friend who years later comes to our aid again, through memory. In some way our whole life prepares us for adversity.

Several times in the book we confront one of the most interesting phenomena I have noted in practice. The same thing that is a comfort to one person may be unhelpful or offensive to another. For example, Lillie, the second cancer survivor profiled in the book, walks by a statue of Christ, looks at the feet and the hands and the wounds, but cannot look into the face and cannot bear the look of compassion. She does not want to see herself as pathetic and in need of pity. In Michael's closing story, he describes the face of a nurse as showing compassion and care. The look of compassion that was a threat to Lillie was a source of comfort and strength for Michael.

The art of medicine consists of finding what is helpful for *this* person at *this* time. This is instructive — not only to the medical professional, but for any who take care of or assist the sick. To know the right thing to say to this person at this time would seem an impossible task. At minimum, *Voices from the Edge* reaffirms the complexity of illness and personality, and it offers the notion that a healer must be flexible and must see each patient and situation as distinct. In this book, doctors who approach each patient with a one-size-fits-all mentality stand out as unhelpful, even hurtful.

Finally, a point of caution. It is one thing to say that in spite of suffering, important lessons are learned. It is another to say that illness occurs to teach or mature someone. Patients have told me consistently that they cannot stand to hear from an outsider that God put this in their life for a reason, even though they may already hold that belief. Though it is true that great discoveries are made in the course of illness, there is in every illness inconsolable suffering, tragic absurdity, a sense that there is no good reason for this, which must be recognized. Cancer patients suffer to the point of terror, rage, and despair. We call it a cancer journey, but we must not forget that it is a journey no one wants to take. The last thing a person drowning in fear and sorrow wants to hear is that there is a jewel of wisdom at the bottom of the pool. We must remember the friends of

Job. For seven days they wept in silence at the sign of his suffering; they were wise, helpful, loving friends. It was when they started rationalizing his suffering that they mortally offended him.

Fortunately, this book does not offer pat, sweeping answers. It does offer possibilities, and it affirms, with the story told by each person, the deep reserve of strength and love that is summoned by adversity.

Patrick W. McLaughlin, MD
Medical Director
Assarian Cancer Center
Providence Cancer Institute
Affiliated with the University of Michigan Medical Center

Emily

I love you all, everything — I can't look at everything
hard enough!

Thornton Wilder, *Our Town*

The "edge" in this book's title refers to a place — not a streetcorner
or clifftop anywhere on this planet, but a place in the minds and
hearts of people who have met death face to face and lived to think
about it. Those who visit this edge gain new vision, a new love for life
in its most brilliant and enchanting detail. They experience clearly
its music and colors and scents and wonders, the daily miracles which
were always there, but which, like most people, they took for granted.

In Thornton Wilder's classic play *Our Town*, Emily's voice is the
voice of a person who has been granted a reprieve from death. Emily
has been to the edge. She has, in fact, crossed it. A young wife, newly
married to her childhood sweetheart, Emily has died in childbirth
and gone to rest in the cemetery with townspeople who have pre-
ceded her in death.

But she cannot rest, cannot let go. Against the entreaties of the
souls who share her new community, she pleads to revisit a day in
her earthly existence. The echo of life is still so fresh in her heart
that she is not ready to let it slip away. Not just yet.

Now back among the living, briefly, she sees the haunting loveli-
ness of the experiences that the living pass through almost without
seeing. The routine events of life — casual meetings, daily frustrations, a careless glance at the setting sun, a quicksilver smile from a
stranger, the flirtations of young love — now have great depth, fresh
layers of meaning.

Emily's newfound appreciation of the joy, pain, and tedium of everyday life is soon tempered by a stinging realization: the living often miss or avoid life. They protect themselves by closing their eyes to the pain of the future. In doing so, they lose sight of the irreplaceable beauty of the present; they pass unseeing within easy reach of the simplest fleeting pleasures.

Emily realizes that her family does not, or cannot, see the magic of the moment. She pleads with them to simply look at one another, to stop and appreciate — and save for all time — the beauty of an instant when all was well with the world:

> . . . just for a moment now we're all together.
> Mama, just for a moment we're happy. Let's look
> at one another!

The truth is this: We are all mortal. We are all in the process of dying, all day, every day. We all live near the edge — but like Emily we don't open our eyes and truly pay attention until we are teetering on the precipice with a clear view of both sides.

The voices in this book are those not of characters in a play but of real people who have been diagnosed with and treated for cancer. They have been to the edge and returned. Some have come back to "normal" life, resolved to endure, to live out the full span of years that they once took for granted, and have put several years between themselves and their diagnosis. Some have returned for only a short stay, and face each day the reality that the next, or the one after that, could be their last. All have returned with a new appetite for life. Their voices ring with their newfound passion — with hope, anger, fear, courage, acceptance, defiance, joy, love, and humor.

Think of those who populate this book as unheralded, unknown, but real (sometimes pseudonymous) citizens of Grover's Corners, people whom Wilder knew in his playwright's soul but didn't write about, people who have suddenly found themselves at the precipice. They have seen what Emily's eyes have seen, learned what her soul has learned, and discovered how unbearably beautiful life becomes in the lengthening shadow of its approaching end. They are not yet ready to follow Emily to her destination; but Emily's words — and the words of Wilder's omniscient narrator — have burned themselves into their hearts:

Emily

It goes so fast. We don't have time to look at one another.

Take me back — up the hill — to my grave. But first: Wait! One more look.

Good-bye. Good-bye world. Good-bye Grover's Corners . . . Mama and Papa. Good-bye to clocks ticking . . . and Mama's sunflowers. And food and coffee. And new-ironed dresses and hot baths . . . and sleeping and waking up. Oh, earth, you're too wonderful for anybody to realize you.

Do any human beings ever realize life while they live it? — every, every minute?

Stage Manager

No.

The saints and poets, maybe — they do some.

TIM HARBOUR, FORTY-FIVE, IS WRITING A BOOK. A good title for Tim's book would be *Seize the Opportunity*, because that's what he does every single day — he seizes the opportunity to live, to love, to share, to teach, to inspire. When he was stricken with a rare form of cancer in 1979, Tim was told he had eighteen months to live. Since then, Tim has been to the edge so many times he can hear the sound of pebbles slipping beneath his feet.

It's not that he fears what he'll find on the other side; it's just that he hasn't finished looking around and absorbing everything this life has to offer. Even more important, he has not finished delivering all his gifts to this life: "I feel I still have a lot to do. We have a reason for being here, and I think part of mine is to be a teacher. Maybe my book will be the start of it.

"There's an insight about living life that comes from facing death. When you face death for as long as I have, it's not that you're not afraid of it anymore, but you learn that it's a part of life, just as important as birth in a way. Cancer gives us these peeks beneath the surface. It opens our eyes to the important things. It's the wake-up call. For an alcoholic, it's bottoming out; for a cancer patient, it's the diagnosis. And some people never get it.

"People always say, 'Well, we're all going to die.' I could punch them in the nose when they say that. Yes, we're all going to die, but if you've been told it's going to be eighteen months from now, that creates a sense of urgency that makes you go at life differently. I sometimes think I wouldn't have had the courage to start my business if I hadn't faced cancer. I might have just plodded along, comfortable in my career as half musician, half engineer and draftsman.

"But I think the interesting side of my story is the other side of it. I've encouraged my wife to write her own book about it. What's it like to sit there for fifteen hours while your husband is undergoing surgery that could mean life or death? And I know that my daughter is a different kind of kid, a very strong person and spiritually deep for a thirteen-year-old, because she's never known a moment in her life when I was well. What's it like to go to school knowing that your father may have months or weeks to live? I think people would like to hear the other side of this."

IN THE COMPANY OF DOCTORS

"I'd had a lump on the right side of my neck, at the base of the skull, since I was twelve. During my high school admission physical, I asked the doctor about it, and he said, 'Ah, it's a cyst. Don't worry about it. If it ever grows, get it looked at.' And it didn't grow, but when I was twenty-four I started getting other lumps around it. I had a biopsy, and it turned out to be a rare type of malignant soft-tissue sarcoma.

"It was certainly a shock to me. The doctors were very negative about my prospects. They were sure I didn't have long to live. They had no idea how to treat it. Radiation wasn't effective, chemotherapy wasn't effective. Surgery was the only treatment."

In many respects, today's research oncologists are a lot like the European explorers of the fifteenth and sixteenth centuries. Their journeys are long and at times tedious, but the lure of discovery is too powerful to resist. The scientists viewed Tim as a virtual continent of unanswered cancer questions. They set out to exploit him to the fullest. But Tim refused to be a passive observer.

"They took out the tumor in December 1979. In January, probably because of some reporting requirement, I got a call from the National Cancer Institute. They were interested in my cancer because it was so rare, and they invited me to come to Bethesda, Maryland. Kind of an all-expenses-paid vacation. I spent three months there. I was evaluated and poked and prodded, and every square inch of my body was examined. My case was presented to

Sarcoma: a malignant tumor growing from connective tissues, such as cartilage, fat, muscle, or bone.

their tumor conference, which involves hundreds of professionals. This conference made its recommendations: exploratory chest surgery to see if my cancer had spread to the lungs, followed by radical neck surgeries on both sides, three months apart. After that, they wanted to do thirty-one radiation treatments to each side of my neck, and then six sessions of chemotherapy — despite the fact that all their scans and X-rays and tests had shown nothing.

"It was mind-boggling. I thought, If the cancer doesn't kill me, the treatment will. There's this incredible medical library at the National Institutes of Health, and there I was with nothing to do each day but undergo a couple of tests. I started poking around, doing a lot of reading, asking questions about alternative therapies and about building up my body's immune system instead of tearing it down.

"When they're saying, 'You go through all this stuff and you've got a 15 percent better chance of living five years,' you go, Wait a minute."

"All the literature was saying that radiation and chemotherapy were not effective against this type of cancer. That scared the hell out of me. It's different if someone says, 'You can do this, and there's a 90 percent chance it's going to be effective.' But when they're saying, 'You go through all this stuff and you've got a 15 percent better chance of living five years,' you go, Wait a minute.

"I especially didn't want to have the radical exploratory surgery on my chest. My preference was just to observe for a few months, then, if we saw any changes, do the surgery. The doctors at NCI didn't like this at all. Apparently they viewed me as some kind of rebel.

"I was in the hospital the night before I was supposed to have the surgery, and I decided at the last minute not to have it. I called the doctor and said, 'I'm not doing it. I just don't feel right about it. I think it makes more sense to keep an eye on it.' Well, the doctors behaved like children. They acted as if I had impugned their integrity. They said, 'If you aren't willing to agree to our recommendations, we're not interested in treating you. Go back to Michigan, find your own doctor, and we'll see you around.'

"Even then, they couldn't just let me go. The chief of clinical surgery came in the next morning and said, 'I want you to know you're making a mistake. If you refuse this surgery, I give you eighteen months to live. You'll probably be well for nine to twelve months, but then you'll start going and you'll go fast.' He said, 'If you live a day longer than eighteen months, I'll be surprised.' He had to get that dig in.

"I was appalled. He had no basis for threatening me — and that's what he was doing, threatening me. And it seemed like he was mostly angry that I had screwed up the operating room schedule. It was an eye-opening experience."

LIMBO

Getting hit with news of accidents, death, or serious disease has a way of transporting you instantly from the land of laundry, car pools, deadlines, and dentist appointments into another dimension. Suddenly you're in the Twilight Zone. Time is distorted, voices are muffled, things look out of place. You're confused and angry because the whole world hasn't joined you on this journey. At first you deal frantically, reflexively, with the crisis. Then everything stops, and doubt and fear begin to creep out of the shadows and threaten you.

"It's like you're floating along on the river, and then you get a diagnosis, and Boom! Suddenly you're in the rapids, and every day it's go here, go there, a doctor's appointment, a scan, an operation, recovery, more tests. It's scary, but you feel like you're going to be okay as long as you're doing something. And then suddenly the rapids spit you out and you're in calm waters again.

"I went back to Michigan, not sure I had done the right thing. I was scared. I thought, Oh my God, what am I going to do now? How am I going to keep this cancer from coming back? I had turned my back on the gods of medicine. These were prestigious people. Most people would be thanking their lucky stars they'd gotten a plane ticket and a hotel room in Bethesda and had the greatest doctors in the world looking at them. Would people think I was nuts?"

CHOOSING TO LIVE

Tim had rejected the only option the researchers had offered him, which appeared to hold more benefits for their research than for his health prospects. It seemed a bleak choice: debilitating surgery or debilitating untreated cancer. He knew his life would never be as it was before, but he was determined that now was not the time for him to die.

"I had gotten this diagnosis in November, and it was almost Easter when I walked out of that hospital. I had lost my job and it was like, how do I get back to living again? And it was definitely a hard thing getting jump-started, almost like I was afraid to start living, as if I was just waiting for the other shoe to drop. You know, when is it going to come back? It was a tough situation. When I was diagnosed, I had no health insurance, so I had to go on state aid — which means I've got to stay unemployed and poor. If I get a job, I risk going three months without coverage."

His future health and his ability to secure employment were of no consequence to one woman who was attracted to his strength, sensitivity, spirit, and determination. "Right in the middle of all this, I met Donna, the girl who would become my wife. We met right before Christmas. I had been diagnosed a month earlier, and we met and had one date, and then I went off to Bethesda for three months. We wrote each other, and so forth, and a year after I got back we got married. And it's such an implausible thing. Who would fall in love with someone who had just been diagnosed with cancer? Donna's an incredible lady."

"It was definitely a hard thing getting jump-started, almost like I was afraid to start living, as if I was just waiting for the other shoe to drop."

Alice in Wonderland asked the Cheshire Cat, "Would you tell me, please, which way I ought to go from here?" To which the cat responded, with a smile: "That depends a good deal on where you want to get to." With Donna in his life, Tim began to understand where it was he wanted to get to. "You know what it really comes down to? Just making a decision. You've got to choose life. You've got to just sit down and say, 'You know what? I am going to live.'

"I'm a very intuitive person, and I have a stubborn and self-reliant nature. The more I thought about it, I knew I had made the right decision. And once I realized that, I found I could move forward.

"I had been doing a lot of research into alternative medicine. The surgeons had removed my tumor, and they believed they had gotten the whole thing. My scans and tests from NIH were clean, except for a shadow in my chest, which is why they wanted to do the exploratory, I guess. I decided that since I didn't have cancer, I would try to stay that way.

"So I dove head first into the world of alternative medicine. I became a vegetarian and started exercising. I read about the power of mind over body. Through my connections in the music business I met an osteopath who specialized in treating cancer with holistic and nutritional natural therapy. I took everything from coffee enemas to calf's liver to handfuls of supplements. I was driven to prove that the physician who had given me eighteen months to live was wrong.

"When I hit eighteen months and one day, Donna and I celebrated. But I was already starting to get lumps in my neck again.

"Two years after I left Bethesda, I had a positive biopsy. So I had the first of my radical neck dissections, on the right side. That was a lot of fun."

Fortunately for Tim, the practitioners he had come to rely on for alternative therapies were not inclined to close the door on

Tim has an appreciation of Western medicine; however, like over one-third of the U.S. population, he looked for alternative ways to improve his health. These readily available practices return a great deal of power to the individual, who is no longer solely a passive recipient. In this respect, such an approach to health care is compelling — particularly noninvasive techniques such as low-fat diets, meditation, guided imagery, biofeedback, moderate exercise, and therapeutic massage. However, because alternative medicine is essentially unregulated, caution must be used when reaching for ingestible over-the-counter therapies or considering experimental treatments.

conventional treatment. "When the osteopath saw the nodes, he said, 'You've got to get these looked at and biopsied.' And while he didn't say, 'Stop the nutritional therapies,' he clearly felt that I would need to see a surgeon. I had read all along that surgery was the only treatment for this kind of cancer."

WEIGHING THE OPTIONS

The next few years of Tim's life became a testament to his indomitable spirit and fierce desire to live. He entered a never-ending cycle of surgery, recovery, and testing every nine to twelve months. The sarcoma kept recurring in the same place. The lymph nodes involved were always on the right side. Since the lymph system is largely divided between left and right, Tim's doctors seemed confident further recurrences would be limited to his right side.

Seven years after the original diagnosis, however, Tim developed a large mass beneath his left ear, which required another neck dissection. And his doctors began to talk about systemic treatment — chemotherapy and radiation.

The specialists, however, said the downside would outweigh the perceived benefits. Besides, Tim had grown tired of the disruptions caused by his cancer and was determined to move on with his life. Although he felt he could tolerate side effects such as fatigue and nausea, he did not want to give cancer any more of his time than was absolutely necessary. He had survived the past; now he was anxious to build a future for Donna and his children. So he opted out of systemic treatment.

"I began to think of it as a chronic disease, like multiple sclerosis or diabetes, something I could live with."

"In retrospect, I might have chosen to try chemo and radiation anyway, but I didn't. By now I had a wife and two daughters, and I had started a business that was doing pretty well. I was living, and these were little bumps along the way, even though some were bigger bumps, like the neck surgeries. I began to think of it as a chronic disease, like multiple sclerosis or diabetes, something I could live with."

JOY, DESPAIR, SALVATION

"For the next six years, I was absolutely clean. I didn't have a single recurrence. No operations, no intervention whatsoever. Even my doctor used the word 'cured.' He said, 'It's been six years. You're out of the woods. That cancer is not coming back.' I can't tell you how good that made me feel.

"In spring 1993, we went to Jamaica with the girls. I went wind surfing and came back with my back hurting. I thought I had pulled a muscle. When I got home, my family doctor looked at it and agreed. But it kept hurting, so I went to an orthopedist, who took an X-ray. I had to tell him my history, of course, and as soon as I said 'sarcoma' he looked at the X-ray and said he wanted to bring in a spine specialist.

"The specialist found a tumor that had already destroyed one of my lumbar vertebrae. It was worse than my original diagnosis. It was like the cruelest joke you could imagine someone playing on you.

"It was devastating. When I was first diagnosed, I was just this starving artist-musician single guy, and now I had all this stuff to lose — wife, family, business. And I had never heard of anybody surviving a spinal metastasis."

Surgeons removed the diseased vertebra and installed metal plates and rods to stabilize his spine. Tim had to wear a plastic full-body brace for nine months. Unable to work, he lost his business. He underwent thirty-two radiation treatments, and on the day he finished those, he had to go to his office, lay off his employees, padlock the doors, and arrange for an auction.

"After I did that, I went home and took my place on the couch. I got up for two reasons — to go to the bathroom, and occasionally to eat. I was thirty-eight, no job, no college degree, dying of cancer, and nobody was going to hire me. I made a depression on that couch for three months, and it got to the point where if the cancer didn't kill me, my wife would.

"Then a couple of things happened. One, a good friend of mine, a wealthy entrepreneur, called me and said, 'I just bought this printing company out of bankruptcy and I need someone who understands digital technology and graphic arts. I'd like you to come and work for me.' This was a major revelation to me, the fact that someone would hire me for my skills and that everything else was irrelevant. It got my butt off the couch.

"The other thing that helped me come out of it was that I was spending a lot more time home with my daughters. I began to realize that I had something to live for, and that if I had come through ten or twelve surgeries and lasted this long, I could make it a while longer."

> "This was a major revelation to me, the fact that someone would hire me for my skills and that everything else was irrelevant."

COMPLICATIONS

The spinal cancer was more aggressive than the original sarcoma, and Tim underwent several operations to remove more vertebrae and an adrenal gland. The frequency and severity of the recurrences, plus the almost continuous cycle of surgery and recovery, made Tim's life more complicated. Not only was cancer continuing to invade his private world with Donna and the children, its physical presence was becoming increasingly apparent to anyone who looked his way.

"Up until then, the cancer wasn't affecting all aspects of my life. By that I mean you couldn't look at me and tell right away that I had cancer. But now I could no longer stand up straight, and I had lost a lot of weight. I developed a chronic anemia that nobody could explain.

"In January '97, I started feeling a lump in my neck again, where the original tumor had been. I had an MRI, and sure enough, I had a mass growing back under the base of my skull against my cervical spine. I saw several different specialists. All of them said it was inoperable and incurable and suggested I get my affairs in order.

"One neurospine specialist at first thought he might do the operation, but decided it was too risky. A surgeon suggested that I had lived eighteen years and should be thankful for it."

BREAKING THE MONOPOLY

From the early days at the National Cancer Institute in Bethesda, Maryland, Tim was an active part of his cancer team. He listened, questioned, researched, challenged, and made it clear that his opinion mattered. Certainly he appreciated the experience and expertise of his physicians. But the final voice, the voice that really mattered, was the one in his heart.

"I've got a great deal of respect for most of the people I've met in medicine over the years. Most of them are dedicated professionals, most are compassionate. But some of them just don't have a clue about people, and I suspect not just in medicine but in life. Why else would a doctor say, 'Now, we know radiation is not effective, and we know chemotherapy is not effective, but why don't we do it anyway?' Can't they understand that when you're faced with a life-or-death decision, you've got to feel right about it?

"Most doctors appreciate a patient who's knowledgeable, who is active in his own treatment. But over the years I've run into these guys who say, 'You wouldn't understand,' and when you push them, they try to dazzle you with some medical gobbledygook, and then you have to say, 'Would you please put that in plain English?'

"Of course, now all you have to do is log onto that beautiful World Wide Web and, guess what? You have more information than they do! Now you can say, 'Hey, have you heard of this clinical trial?' I don't know if doctors like it or not, but for a long time people just didn't ask questions because they were worried about offending their physician. It was a different world back then. Doctors did not always appreciate a patient challenging a recommendation.

"I went to this guy who is supposedly the preeminent sarcoma specialist in the country. During my first consultation with him, he asked me if I had taken a particular alternative medicine. I admitted I had. He flew off the handle, got wildly angry, and refused to take my case. Now, most doctors would say, 'Hey, if it's not hurting, why not?' After all, they've shown there can be a very powerful effect if the patient believes it's helping."

A TRIP TO THE SUMMIT

The doctor's advice to get his affairs in order just made Tim mad. He had heard this advice before and his reaction was the same now as it was then: he wasn't about to give up. He sought more opinions, including one from the surgeon who had done his spine surgeries. The surgeon referred Tim to a friend and colleague at the Mayo Clinic. Three days later Tim was at the world-famous clinic in Rochester, Minnesota, undergoing a whirlwind of consultations.

"An incredible place," says Tim. "Very different from NCI or any other place. I had never been in a facility that was so patient-centered. Each examination room has a couch and a little private area where you can dress, and they don't make you walk through a crowded waiting room with your butt hanging out of the hospital gown.

"A team of surgeons got the tumor out, stabilized my spine with screws and rods, and screwed my skull to my cervical spine so I'd be able to hold my head up. The operation took sixteen hours. I spent three months in halo traction. And I lost weight. I was a six-foot, 170-pound man when I first got the spine cancer. After the Mayo operation I was down to 120 pounds. I can't gain the weight back. I have difficulty swallowing, and it takes me two or three times as long as the average person to eat a meal. It's hard for me to drive, because I can't move my head up or down, left or right. I have difficulty walking. I'm in fairly severe chronic pain. I've had to quit my job and go on Social Security disability. I was lucky that I had private disability insurance through my friend's company, too."

Chronic disease often robs its victims of the simple pleasures of life. The pain, the struggle, the fear of an early demise are overshadowed by the missed enjoyment of ordinary events. When did my child learn to tie her shoes? Where was I when he caught his first baseball? Did I really miss her high school graduation? How could I not have noticed those beautiful wildflowers that have always grown by the side of the road?

"Over the years I've gone through this grieving process for each thing. I used to be able to pick up my daughter and bounce her; I can't do that anymore. I liked being the family breadwinner, simply getting up and going to work.

"So I decided if I couldn't work anymore, I would write a book. I had a friend, a literature professor at Wayne State, who had been encouraging me for years. I started writing, and I joined a writers' group. And it's going well."

A Dream Fulfilled

Trips to the edge make you anxious to fast-forward to the future. You want to get to the good parts now in case there is no later — even if it's just for a quick glance.

"We moved down to Florida and built a house after the Mayo operation. Beautiful house, right on the beach. We've always loved the ocean, and we just decided that regardless of what happened we would take advantage of the chance to do it now, as opposed to when I'm dead.

"But the cancer recurred on my spine, so I had to go back to Michigan for another operation. I recovered, we went back to Florida, and within a month I was back in Michigan again. The tumors in my spine were starting to paralyze me.

"Finally I agreed to have chemotherapy in Florida. In nineteen years of treatment, I'd never had chemo. And that was an experience. I had a pretty tough time with it. I tried to psych myself up for it, to view it as an ally instead of an enemy. But it was tough. I lost more weight, and all of my hair.

"We moved back to Michigan. I started in a clinical trial of a vaccine grown from my tumor, but

> *"We should write because it is human nature to write. Writing claims our world. It makes it directly and specifically our own. We should write because humans are spiritual beings and writing is a powerful form of prayer and meditation, connecting us both to our own insights and to a higher and deeper level of inner guidance."*
>
> — Julia Cameron,
> *The Right to Write*

the cancer came back on my spine, and this time my surgeon was not enthusiastic about doing more surgery. And, in fact, I wasn't either. It was getting ridiculous. It used to be surgery would buy me a year, year and a half. Now it was surgery every few weeks.

"I was ready to give up. The chemo failed, radiation failed, the vaccine failed. There really weren't any options left.

"Donna and I talked about it. Along toward Christmas I decided I would try one more time. I had done some research on the Internet and found that they were starting some trials using thalidomide to treat sarcomas. I decided to have the surgery so I could start with a clean slate. I got on the thalidomide study four weeks later, but I have since had to quit taking it due to peripheral neuropathy."

THE ESSENTIAL TIM

When you talk with Tim, you are struck by his intelligence, his profound love for his family, and his firm understanding that he is *not* his cancer, not just his body. His spirit transcends all the pushing, prodding, dissecting, radiating, and poisoning he has been subjected to over all these years.

"I'm a deeply spiritual person, but I'm not very religious, so I'm not one of those people who will tell you, 'God got me through this.' It was nothing more than a really deep love of life and a fierce desire to keep living it, to get my tail up and go again each time I get knocked down.

Chemotherapy is the treatment or control of cancer using anticancer drugs: highly toxic medications that destroy cancer cells by interfering with their growth or preventing their reproduction. Chemo is most effective against rapidly reproducing cells — both good and bad cells. Therefore, healthy cells in the body that divide rapidly are most affected. Some of those cells that normally divide rapidly are hair cells, bone marrow cells, and the cells lining the mouth and other parts of the intestinal tract. As a result, people on chemotherapy may develop bone marrow depression, lose their hair, and get mouth sores.

"I love people, and I love watching my daughters grow. This may sound like I'm oversimplifying life, but the beginning and end of the whole thing is that we're here to love and be loved."

C. S. Lewis was once asked, "Why should the righteous suffer?" "Why not?" he replied. "They're the only ones that can handle it."

I asked Tim, "When you're alone in the middle of the night with only your thoughts, what gives you the strength to face each day knowing that there will be obstacles and pain?" He replied, "I don't mean to sound corny or trite, but the fact is, I love life. I love everything about it, and I am not ready to give it up."

Tim's voice is one of hope, perseverance, and commitment to family and the joys of life. In his world there is no time for whining, self-pity, or surrender. It's been twenty-one years since that one doctor in Bethesda told him he had eighteen months to live. Twenty-one years to shape a life based on his interpretation of what was possible — not someone else's. Twenty-one years to spend with his family and friends. Twenty-one years of giving and sharing.

The challenge for the rest of us is to know Tim's joy without having to feel Tim's pain. As Emily might have asked in Our Town: Can we do it? Can we truly appreciate what we have without having to look over the edge? Can we remember to hold our gaze on today's sunset without a constant reminder that tomorrow's performance may occur without us? Can we face an inconvenience or annoyance without responding as though to a full-blown disaster? Can we pause long enough to really look at the faces of those we love instead of just stealing glances? Perhaps not to the same extent as Emily or Tim, but we can certainly try. We can accept Tim's gift — the sharing of his journey — and return the offering by resolving to walk just a little bit slower; to smile just a little bit more; and to complain just a little bit less.

We must recognize the power of our two voices: the voice we use to connect with those around us and, more important, the inner voice that whispers in the middle of the night so that only we can hear.

2

The Voice of Humor

LILLIE SHOCKNEY, FORTY-SIX, HAS BEEN TO THE EDGE TWICE. Both times, she pondered the mysteries of the other side and walked away with renewed strength, a determination to live a full and happy life, and a deep desire to help others.

Not to mention her wonderful sense of humor. Having dinner with her at her favorite Seattle restaurant, I am at her mercy. We are both drawing stares from the other diners. And what are we laughing about? Cancer.

Lillie, a registered nurse, is the director of education and outreach at the Johns Hopkins Breast Center. She has also been diagnosed twice with breast cancer and, in two operations three years apart, had both of her breasts removed. To increase her chances of detecting any recurrence, Lillie has elected not to have reconstructive surgery. Instead, she wears two prostheses. She has named them Bobbie Sue and Betty Boob.

"A very dear friend of mine sent me a Christmas gift: stick-on nipples," says Lillie. "They're made of silicone, but they didn't come with instructions or adhesives. My husband suggested, 'Put a few drops of water on the back and maybe it will stick to your prosthesis.' I tried this, and it seemed to work. Why I thought my husband was an expert in the use of stick-on nipples remains a mystery to me.

"I had to give a formal presentation at work, so I decided to take

Cancer is obviously not a subject to be taken lightly, but without the power of humor, those on the edge in their battle with cancer will lose. With laughter, you reduce the power of the disease to kill your spirit, and maybe, just maybe, your body as well. Just ask Lillie.

my new nipples for a test drive. I felt very risqué. I had on a silk shell, and I looked in the mirror and thought, They're very subtle, but oh yes, I can see them. I thought this was the best thing since sliced bread.

"My presentation went well. It was on how we have improved surgical care for women diagnosed with breast cancer. I had slides, so I was doing a lot of pointing and arm waving. Afterward, I sat down next to a male colleague I hadn't seen for a year. It was hot, so I took off my jacket. I felt very pleased with myself in my sleeveless silk shell.

"Coming around the table on a beautiful china plate were these Pepperidge Farm cookies. I reached over to take the plate from my colleague. Then I looked down at my little dessert plate, where I was supposed to place my cookie. There was already a cookie on it.

"It was my left nipple.

"So I'm sitting there, holding this heavy dessert plate, and the man looks at my plate and says, 'Oh, I didn't see they had those thin wafer cookies. That's my favorite! Darn, it looks like you got the last one.'

"'It's my favorite too,' I said. 'I'm going to save it for later.' In a flash, I grabbed the nipple and shoved it in my pocket. He looked at me like I was crazy.

"My husband said later it was a good thing I grabbed it first. 'That man would still be chewing,' he said."

A SERIOUS WOMAN, LAUGHING

We discuss many things — building support groups, using the Internet to deliver health information, the latest treatments for a variety of cancers, the mind-body-spirit connection, the importance of early detection, the lifesaving advantage of quick interventions. But Lillie's irreverent humor helps vanquish the three-headed monster — fear, pain, and doubt — that threatens to dominate the life of a cancer patient. Her approach to illness, death, and living helps her take back some of the control, to recognize that, yes, there are needles, nausea, worry, pain, and fear, but also joy, laughter, hope, shared experiences — and, of course, the occasional platter of thin wafer cookies.

Standing just a little over five feet tall, Lillie is a mixture of intelligence, wit, compassion, vulnerability, and strength. Where did she get her "true grit," her assertive presence in the face of the "C" word? Lillie draws some of this strength from her early years growing up on a Maryland dairy farm. There, at the tender age of six, she began to assume the responsibility for many of the chores, including milking the cows.

"We milked them every morning, we milked them every evening, and we had to keep the barn clean, because you never knew when the inspector might show up. That meant before school, and just as soon as school was over, you had a date with the cows.

"On Saturday, we were out working in the barn or running behind a tractor with a wagon picking up bales of straw or bales of hay, or going out to do something with alfalfa. There was never much time for anything else, including making friends."

As Lillie tells it, her spartan childhood was relieved by a friendship with an older woman who taught her lessons that Lillie, years later, would pass on to thousands of other women. This particular woman, this friend, this mentor was affectionately called Miss Bertha.

"Bertha was actually my mother's friend," says Lillie, "but she called me her 'borrowed daughter.' She was my best friend."

WHISPERS

When Lillie was twelve, Miss Bertha was diagnosed with breast cancer. Now, keep in mind that in the late 1960s, the word "cancer" was often only whispered and never discussed openly in

Lillie's strength of character is something I haven't seen since my year in sixth grade at Saints Peter & Paul School in Jamestown, New York, with Sister Mary Ada, whose tales of religious virtue could also inspire. Where Lillie relies on the sturdy and wonderful resonance of her voice for effect, Sister Ada mesmerized and controlled her classroom audience with a quiet, reverent tone — a whisper that filled the room with wondrous yarns about Christian heroes. Like Lillie, Sister Ada was kind — gentle and encouraging to pupils who were slow to understand the lessons, sensitive and sympathetic with the poor kids.

polite company, and you most assuredly didn't hear the word "breast" unless you were talking to your doctor or learning about "the facts" from your mother.

"I didn't know if people's teeth would fall out or their eyeballs would melt or what," Lillie said. "It was forbidden to mention those words in a public place. But, I noticed, even as a youngster, you couldn't bring it up even in the privacy of your own home. You could say 'She's ill,' or 'She has a female problem,' but beyond that, you couldn't say much."

As Lillie later found out, the doctor told Bertha that the softball-sized lump in her breast was advanced cancer that had metastasized to her ribs, her liver, and her lungs. He was blunt: no hope. It meant a complete removal of the breast and the surrounding muscle tissue, full-body radiation, and chemotherapy. Having skipped the med-school class on bedside manner, the doctor told her that she really needn't concern herself about the length of treatment. He said, "You're not going to be alive to see the end of treatment, because you're going to be dead within five months."

Lillie remembers how Miss Bertha broke the news to her: "'The doctor says I'm going to die. I told him I'm not going to do any such thing. He said to go home and get my affairs in order, and I said, "I don't have time to do that; I'm too busy living." Then I said to him, 'I've made a list of things I'm going to do before I leave this world. And my first goal, Mister, is to outlive you!'"

"I asked her, 'How do you know, Miss Bertha?' She said,

There was little scientific knowledge connecting laughter to health and healing in 1967, when Bertha, a psychologist, promised to beat cancer with laughter. But today we know that laughter is good medicine. Scientific studies have shown that a good belly laugh can, among other benefits, lower blood pressure and release endorphins — chemicals in the brain that ease pain and make you feel good. Laughter is also thought to improve circulation, stimulate the nervous system, strengthen the heart, and enhance the immune system. It relieves pent-up tension, and by doing so, defends against stress.

'Because I want to that badly. I believe in optimism. I believe what the doctor says about the medical treatment, and I want to be aggressive in combating this disease, but I'm also going to find something to laugh about every day to help build my immune system.'

"When I tried to talk about Miss Bertha with my mother, all she could say was, 'I'm so afraid we're going to lose Miss Bertha.' 'But she says we aren't going to,' I replied. And my mother said, 'I can't talk about it.'

"I had just gotten my own breasts. I remember feeling them and wondering, Are these going to be trouble?"

Miss Bertha lived another twenty-one years. What she did during that time helped prepare Lillie for what was to come. Besides giving her an early primer on the psychology and physiology of breast cancer, Miss Bertha was a role model who faced bitter adversity head-on while she squeezed out every drop of the sweet juice that life had to offer.

In Rochester, New York, Miss Bertha had a friend, Lena, who would come to visit her quite often. Lena had had bilateral mastectomies done two years before Miss Bertha. At a time when there were virtually no formal support groups, these women provided comfort to one another. They also let young Lillie hear the candid details of their experiences with breast cancer. Miss Bertha used to tell Lillie, "You say you want to be a nurse someday, so it's important that you hear these things."

Bertha also said something ironically prophetic shortly before she died. She told Lillie, "I'm so thankful you've always been my 'borrowed' daughter and not my daughter by blood. I wouldn't want to think that I would have run the risk of passing this disease on to you."

The most powerful risk factors are genetic: Do you have a family history of the disease? Does your mother, father, sister, brother, son, or daughter (first-degree relative) have breast cancer? Does your aunt, uncle, grandfather, or grandmother (second-degree relative) have breast cancer? Is there an inherited genetic mutation for breast cancer in your family? Do you have the gene?

THE SHOCK OF DISCOVERY

Five years after Miss Bertha died, Lillie was diagnosed with first-stage cancer in her left breast. She was thirty-eight.

Lillie had a history of benign cysts, and she was having a routine needle biopsy of yet another one in her right breast. The doctor ordered a baseline mammogram of her left breast. Then he delivered some startling news: "Though there is no palpable lump in your left breast, you do have a small spot that warrants a biopsy."

A few days later, a surgeon performing a biopsy under local anesthetic said, "Your mammogram was deceptive about how diseased your breast really is." And he said, "I'm going to remove a much larger section of tissue than I had planned. This tissue is very gray." And he said, "I'm going to be out of town for five days. I would like to be the one to personally review your pathology report with you rather than one of my partners. Are you going to be okay waiting?" And Lillie said, "Sure."

"I was like, Let's function in the land of denial," says Lillie. "Normally I would have had to wait only two days. If the news were good, one of his partners could have told me. Heck, a housekeeper could have told me! But I thought, It's benign, so I'm not going to worry about it.

"I'm a nurse, so I should have known better, but two days later, at work, I went to the computer, pulled up my report, and read the word 'cancer' twelve times. And I saw the Grim Reaper staring at me out of that screen."

Devastated, Lillie ran toward the exit, as though by running fast enough she could escape what seemed to be a death sentence. "There was a family in the hallway. They were laughing, feeling good about something. I stopped and

Breast cancer is the most common cancer in women, and is second only to lung cancer as a cause of cancer deaths. The American Cancer Society estimates that approximately 175,000 new cases were diagnosed in women in 1999. Despite the fact that 43,300 women were expected to die of the disease in 1999, the mortality rate for breast cancer is falling — due, experts believe, to early detection and improved treatment.

looked at them and thought, How can you be laughing? I have breast cancer!

"To reach the door, I had to pass by the statue of Christ. I stopped. I looked at his hands, I looked at his feet. But I couldn't look at his eyes. I thought, I can't look at your face right now; I'll have to see if I can look at it in the morning. I knew that his expression would be filled either with compassion or pity and, at the moment, I knew that either one of those looks might well trigger hysteria. I could not handle that.

"I thought about Miss Bertha, but all I could think was, She's gone, she's gone!"

THE COMFORT OF MEMORY

Later, after the initial shock had worn off, Lillie's thoughts again came around to Miss Bertha, and this time she took comfort in her late friend's strength. "Bertha was the kind of person who shaped her own world to her needs. Her husband was inattentive; she found friendship elsewhere. The doctors gave her no hope, so she created her own.

"Bertha made her own fun. I remember one particular Saturday when Bertha had promised to take me walking on the beach. The day came, and it was pouring rain. When I got to her house, I said, "I guess we aren't going walking.' 'Why not?' she said. 'Well, it's raining.' 'So it is.' She handed me a slicker, and we walked along the beach picking up these beautiful pieces of glass that had been smoothed by the surf. After a bit she raised her face to the sky. 'Feel the rain on your face,' she said. 'Taste the rain in your mouth.' That was the nicest beach walk. I'll never forget it.

"Bertha decided that, no matter what she was told, she was going to live. So why should I let anybody persuade me otherwise?"

"Bertha decided that, no matter what she was told, she was going to live. So why should I let anybody persuade me otherwise? If Bertha could make her own fun, find her own hope — if she could prove the experts wrong — why shouldn't I?"

Lillie understood that where others saw disappointment, Bertha grabbed opportunity. Where others saw barriers, Bertha found stepping stones. Where others saw glass, Bertha discovered rare jewels. When others felt drenched and cold, Bertha felt refreshed and renewed. But Bertha did much more than this. She saw a lost little girl who needed a friend, and she took her in. She shared walks and laughter as well as tragedy and sorrow. She taught Lillie that although a certain amount of pain is inevitable in life, suffering is an option. We can feel and even embrace the pain, but we need to let the suffering go. Pain strikes a chord that, in time, may resonate with joy. Suffering, on the other hand, simply sits and selfishly steals your precious energy without thought of return. One is a wondrous part of the universe; the other is man-made and seeks only to satisfy its insatiable appetite and leave you empty. Cry and feel the pain, and then let the suffering find somewhere else to feed.

To this day, when Lillie talks about Miss Bertha, you will catch her eyes focusing on a scene painted vividly in her memory: the two of them skipping down Fifth Avenue after watching a show at Radio City Music Hall, Lillie dressed in her best little kid outfit, Miss Bertha in her mink — both wearing Keds tennis shoes that they bought the day before at Macy's. Or she's back on Miss Bertha's thirteen-foot sailboat, listening to the waves gently applauding as they drift across Chesapeake Bay.

DELIVERING BAD NEWS

After discovering that she had cancer, Lillie did not remember much about the ride home. "But I did hold onto a very important thought: I had something Bertha didn't have — my wise, wonderful, supportive husband, Al, loving parents, and my delightful twelve-year-old daughter, Laura — yep, same age as I was when Miss Bertha got cancer.

"I knew Al wouldn't be home until eleven, nearly four hours later, and I didn't want Laura to know yet. Then I began to think, Who will raise her? How will my husband get through this? How will I tell him? I practiced telling him in front of the mirror. I was going to explain how Mom had been calling me, asking about the biopsy results, and I was sure it would be good news, so I had looked up the report myself instead of waiting for the doctor to return.

"But it didn't work out that way. When my husband arrived, I met him at the door and said, 'Al, I have breast cancer.' 'Okay,' he said. 'Okay. We don't know how bad it is, but that's okay. I don't care if it's the worst it can be, because I know something. I know you. There is no one on this earth with more of a zest for living and stronger willpower than you. We're going to beat this.' And to this day he hasn't wavered.

"For three days I kept the news from my daughter. She kept asking, 'Is anything wrong? Everybody's being so quiet.' I'd say, 'No, everything's fine.' But she knew something was wrong. Kids know.

"When I broke the news to her, I put myself in Miss Bertha's place. I knew there were two questions she would ask, because most children in that situation ask them. She asked, 'Mommy, are you going to die?' I told her, 'No, I think I'm going to be fine. Now, that may change, but I don't think so. After all, you're about to turn thirteen. Do you think God would leave you with Daddy to take you through your teenage years alone?' And she said, 'No, Daddy's hair is already white and that would make it all fall out!'

"Then she asked me a question that a typical kid would think, but rarely ask, because it's too frightening: 'Did you get breast cancer

When there's trouble in the house — any trouble — children Laura's age, and even younger, know that something is not right. Mom and Dad look at each other differently; the whispers are deafening; and the secret code is easily broken or, worse, misinterpreted. "Are you and Mom getting a divorce? Are we poor? Do we have to move? Am I in trouble? Did Dad lose his job? Is somebody going to die?" These are only some of the questions that run through a child's mind. Using appropriate language, let your children know the truth if you find yourself on the edge — the sooner the better. After all, if it impacts their lives, they have a right to know. They're going to find out eventually, and you'll feel better for telling them.

because you had me?' I assured her that was certainly not the case —
that it wasn't anybody's fault at all, it was just something that happens sometimes and nobody knows why.

"Her next question came out of left field, but it helped me find
my sense of humor instantly. She asked, 'Will the doctor let you bring
your breast home to keep?' She said, 'After all, it isn't his, it's yours.
You can put it in Daddy's big pickle jar and keep it on the mantle downstairs, and when you're sad you can go down and look at it.' I said to
my husband, 'How would that look? On the mantle, we've got your
bluefish, your deer head, and over here, my 44D in a pickle jar.' He
said, 'I guess I'd have to go back to Sam's Club and get a bigger
pickle jar!'"

Laura's curiosity grew and grew. 'Will the doctor take your right
breast and move it to the middle? If he doesn't, you're going to lean
to the right when you walk.' I said, 'I'm going to be wearing a bra with
a pocket in it to hold a breast prosthesis. It will look like my breast,
even though it isn't actually attached to me.' She said, 'Oh! A bra
with a pocket! What a clever thing! You always worry when you go to
the ATM bank machine that somebody's going to steal your money.
You could put it in that pocket and no one could get it.' I said, 'Well,
that's true, but I go from there to the grocery store, and when it's
time to pay the bill, we could have a problem.' And my husband said,
'I think she gave you an excellent recommendation. I hate waiting
in those long lines with you at the grocery store. You could start
getting your money out and we could make an express line wherever
we want to.'

"My daughter had found *our* sense of humor and lost most of
her fear."

WHO NEEDS TO KNOW?

Later, Lillie asked Al whether she should keep her mastectomy a
private matter or go public. "Al told me, 'If you make other people
aware that this happened to you, maybe they'll get a mammogram.'
So, after thinking it over, I told my staff, and soon all 16,000 people
at the institution knew that Lillie Shockney had breast cancer.

"People would see me in the hallway and say, 'I heard you were ill, but it must be a mistake. You look fine.' And I'd say, 'Well, I have breast cancer, but I feel fine.'

"I called the radiology department and said, 'You may want to extend your mammography hours, because I think you're going to have a lot of employees as patients.' And they sure did. Foxhole religion kicked in, and women who had never before had a mammogram came in and got one. Al was right."

It is estimated that one woman in eight is at risk of developing breast cancer during her lifetime. To put that frightening statistic in perspective, it's helpful to know that by "lifetime," statisticians mean over the course of ninety-five years. Understanding what "risk" means is important. Risk is a statistical calculation based on the incidence of disease in a group of people who have a specific trait compared with a group of people who are similar but do not have that trait. Most experts believe that knowing the probability of developing breast cancer for a particular age group gives a more realistic picture of one's own odds. Here is the breast cancer risk by age:

Chances of Developing Breast Cancer

by age 25: 1 in 19,608
by age 30: 1 in 2,525
by age 35: 1 in 622
by age 40: 1 in 217
by age 45: 1 in 93
by age 50: 1 in 50
by age 55: 1 in 33
by age 60: 1 in 24
by age 65: 1 in 17
by age 70: 1 in 14
by age 75: 1 in 11
by age 80: 1 in 10
by age 85: 1 in 9
ever: 1 in 8

Source: NCI Surveillance Program

ROUND TWO

One year after her first mastectomy, Lillie found a lump in her right breast and knew it wasn't a cyst. She underwent a lumpectomy to remove a large, rapidly growing benign mass. Just ten month later, when her next mammogram was done, she got bad news again — her other breast was diseased and needed to be removed.

To nobody's surprise, Lillie responded with an even stronger commitment to increase awareness and help others. She wrote a book, *Breast Cancer Survivor's Club;* she became a motivational speaker; and she cofounded "Mothers with Daughters with Breast Cancer" — an organization dedicated to providing information about breast cancer, as well as tips for mothers on how to support daughters (borrowed or blood) who are diagnosed with the disease. In addition, Lillie commits endless hours simply being there for people. She has reached out and touched hundreds of thousands with her message and example.

Recently, Lillie and I were trading e-mail about this book when she confided that she had just received a call from someone at Johns Hopkins asking her to talk with a woman in California who had just received some very bad news. "'Work your wonderful magic and help this woman for me, please,' is what he said to me.

"I told him I didn't have any magic, but he said, 'The sound of your voice is magic — you just don't know it yet.'

"I hope I can help this woman. She apparently needs to achieve closure in her life, and quite soon. These are the ones that I cry myself to sleep about when I'm through."

LEAVE 'EM LAUGHING

We have already made a spectacle of ourselves in our fancy Seattle restaurant, and the waiter and half the patrons are eyeing us suspiciously. Then Lillie tells the story that leads to our total collapse, the hasty delivery of our check, and an icy "Have a nice evening!"

"After Miss Bertha's friend Lena had her bilateral mastectomy, she realized that she could now be whatever bra size she wanted. She was a gymnastics teacher — but not your typical gymnastics teacher, because she was six feet tall and large-breasted. She tried to wear breast prostheses, but this was long before there were mastectomy bras with pockets to keep them secure. She discovered the hard way that doing cartwheels in public caused these objects to become airborne and created quite a stir.

"So she bought an inflatable bra and was very happy with it for a time. It was light in weight and allowed her to do the gymnastics routines that she enjoyed. One day she was flying out of town to visit a family member and, as always, had on her inflatable bra — inflated to the max, because she had been a buxom woman.

"There are lots of signs in an airplane telling you what to do and what not to do. You know, signs that tell you where the exits are, signs that tell you not to smoke. But there are no signs that say, 'Persons wearing inflatable bras must deflate them before takeoff.'

"They had been airborne about fifteen minutes, and she was having a conversation with the man in the seat next to her, when suddenly her chest started vibrating. He looked at her chest, and she looked at her chest, and just as the thought occurred to her to run to the back of the plane, POW! POW! her bra exploded.

"She scurried to the restroom, removed her sweater and turtleneck, and assessed the damage. Major blowouts, right through the nipples. She used tissues to fill what atmospheric pressure had deflated, stitched the nipples shut with her sewing kit, reassembled herself, and decided to go back to her seat and make believe nothing had happened.

"She attempted to pick up the conversation where she had left off, but while she was in the bathroom, the man sitting next to her had lost his peripheral vision and gone deaf. He wouldn't look at her or listen to her. She sat there giggling for the remainder of the flight. Another day in the life of a breast cancer survivor!"

Oh, one last thing. Remember Betty Boob and Bobbie Sue? Well, Lillie's goal is to learn ventriloquism so that she can have Betty Boob and Bobbie Sue deliver health messages about the importance of breast self-examination and mammography.

How would you like to be sitting next to her on an airplane when she's rehearsing?

"You have cancer." Not once but twice Lillie had to confront the fears, concerns, and challenges that come packaged with those words. She could have shaken her fist at God, retreated into a shell of self-pity, protected her privacy, or simply turned a blind eye to the reality of the disease. She could have, but she didn't. With the spirit of Miss Bertha and a profound love for life, she turned personal adversity into something wonderful and meaningful for thousands of people — people with and without cancer. Of course Lillie cried, was afraid, became self-absorbed, and had moments of intense doubt, but these were only moments. Each time, she picked herself up and marched ahead as if to say, "Okay, life, let's see what's around the next corner!" And as she peeked around that next corner, it was always with a sense of optimism, even humor — but not dread. She has a framed parchment in her computer room that she reads every night. It says, "Laughter is God's hand on the shoulder of a troubled world." It is one of the things that gets her through.

Lillie says, "I was given an extraordinary gift — the gift of knowing why I got cancer. I don't mean I know what caused it, but I do know why it happened. It happened so that I could combine my nursing skills with my personal experience as a patient and become the lifeline for other women who end up walking in my shoes — or wearing my bra."

For most women, Lillie is an image of hope, of survivorship; for others, for breast cancer patients who cannot become long-term survivors, she's the one to help them achieve closure with themselves and with their families. But she teaches them all how to live on in memory, how to instill their values into their children before they go, and how to be remembered for those values and special qualities for many years to come. It is a taxing job, but it's her personal mission, and she has chosen to devote her professional and personal time to this cause.

At various times in our lives, we all encounter cancers of one kind or another: decaying friendships, a job that makes days feel like weeks, bills that grow like weeds, missed opportunities, lost love, the pain of losing our parents — or worse, our children — and the awareness of good times passing too quickly. Although painful and at times devastating, troubles remind us that we are still alive and provide a backdrop of contrast that elevates our joys, clarifies our blessings, and tempers our boasts. Of course, these cancers can also send us into permanent hiding, lead to terminal bitterness, and numb all sense of joy. The beauty is that we control the medicine that leads to recovery. Whether we administer it or not is up to us.

3

The Voice of Discovery

LOU DESFOSSES IS A SIXTY-TWO-YEAR-OLD UNIVERSITY PROFESSOR with a long and distinguished career. "I did all the typical academic things. I wrote, I published, I taught, I did a lot of consulting in the United States and Europe. I was in a Fulbright program that required working with companies in Hungary with a concentration in the cities of Budapest and Miskolc, helping them learn the Western way of doing business. I was making a contribution, and I felt good about that.

"Now, looking back on it, if I had a choice between getting another grant or living longer, having better relationships with family and friends, there would be no question. I would stay with living longer, getting more out of life. I've got a twenty-something-page résumé that I would gladly trade for some relief from this cancer."

BAD ADVICE

Lou's story is filled with irony, tragedy, and hope. He was wise enough to follow the advice of his wife. He also followed the advice of his physician — which, in this case, was a mistake.

"What happened was that my wife had a cancerous polyp in her colon. They caught it in time, and there's no further trace of cancer, but she was much exercised about it. She told me, 'At your age you ought to be getting a colonoscopy.'

"I was motivated enough to go to my doctor and ask for a colonoscopy. He gave me an office digital. You know how useless that is; an office digital normally picks up maybe 2 to 4 percent of colon cancers. He felt around, checked my prostate, gave me the quick-strip hemoccult, and said, 'You're fine. Don't worry about a thing.' I said, 'I'd really like to have a colonoscopy, just to be sure.' He said, 'Well, these tests can be dangerous; there's a danger of perforation. We can't be just prescribing tests when they are unnecessary.' This, in spite of the National Cancer Institute's well-publicized recommendation for colonoscopy or sigmoidoscopy every three to five years beginning at age fifty.

"This happened four times. Every year I'd come back and ask for a colonoscopy, partly because several of my friends were dying of colon cancer. On the fourth visit, I had some symptoms. Again I asked for a colonoscopy. The doctor went through the usual digital exam and said I didn't need it. I said, 'Look, either prescribe it, refer me, or I'm going to find a doctor who will.' Finally he agreed to it.

"After the colonoscopy, one look at the gastroenterologist's face told me I was in deep trouble. I had a fairly large polyp that had to be taken out.

Colonoscope: *an instrument similar in function to a sigmoidoscope but much longer, in most cases enabling the doctor to see the lining of the entire colon.*

Double contrast barium enema: *a procedure in which barium sulfate, a chalky substance, is injected through the anus to partially fill and open up the colon. When the colon is about half-full of barium, the patient is turned on the x-ray table so the barium spreads throughout the colon. Then air is injected to cause the colon to expand, providing better X-ray images.*

Fecal occult blood test ("quick strip hemoccult"): *a test used to find occult (hidden) blood in feces. Blood vessels at the surface of colorectal adenomas or cancers are often fragile and easily damaged by the passage of feces.*

Rectal examination: *an examination in which the doctor, wearing thin gloves, puts a greased finger into the rectum and gently feels for lumps.*

Sigmoidoscope: *a slender, flexible, hollow, lighted tube about the thickness of a finger. It is connected to a video camera and video display monitor and inserted through the rectum up into the colon. This allows the doctor to look at the inside of the rectum and part of the colon for cancer or for polyps. Because it is only 60 centimeters (around 2 feet) long, the doctor is able to see only about half of the colon.*

"The surgeon who was to do the operation asked me, 'Why didn't you come earlier? Why weren't you tested?' I told him about the last four years — how I had asked for a colonoscopy and was told that it wasn't necessary. He said, 'These guys will never learn. Every year the NCI and all the other cancer organizations send out their warnings and guidelines, and nobody listens to them.'

"I now have a colostomy and all the problems associated with that, and a death sentence I have to live with."

FACING REALITY

Lou's colonoscopy was followed by a CAT scan at a local hospital. The results at first seemed to indicate that the cancer had not spread, but the surgeon checked manually during the operation and found cause for alarm. "He said, 'I don't know how to explain this, but you have a big problem here. The cancer has spread to your liver.' As it turned out, the CAT scan was done on an older, underpowered machine. Another scan, using a more advanced machine, showed at least a dozen tumors, some of considerable size.

Cancer of the colon: *a common form of cancer in which malignant cells are found in the tissues of the colon. The colon is part of the body's digestive system. The purpose of the digestive system is to gather nutrients (vitamins, minerals, carbohydrates, fats, proteins, and water) from the foods eaten and to store the waste until it passes out of the body. The digestive system is made up of the esophagus, stomach, and the small and large intestines. The last six feet of intestine is called the large bowel or colon.*

Colostomy: *a surgical operation that creates an artificial anus through an opening made in the abdomen from the colon.*

Polyp: *a small, stalk-shaped growth sticking out from the skin or from a mucous membrane. Polyps are mostly benign, but some become malignant.*

Stage four: *a diagnosis in which the cancer has spread completely through the wall of the colon or rectum into nearby tissues or organs.*

"At that point I broke down, because the reality was obvious and unavoidable. I couldn't stop crying. It was so overwhelming. My wife got one of the hospital religious counselors to talk to me. He came into the room, and I was crying, and he said, 'Tell me about the problem.' I told him I had just found out I had cancer in my liver and the talk was about how much time I had left. And I started to cry, and he started to cry. It turned out he had cancer of the liver that he thought had been cured but had come back, and it didn't look good for him either. Fortunately, his story had a happy ending. Although pressed for another liver resection by his surgeons, he refused. After a personal conversation with God that took place as he worked in his garden, he came to the realization, with the help of God, that the operation was unnecessary. Today he is in complete remission."

*As a person in his sixties,
Lou clearly qualified for a colonoscopy or the double
contrast barium enema. Had he had either of these, the story might well
have been different. Why did Lou wait so long to confront the doctor? Why didn't he
get a second opinion early in the game? Unlike most men, he stated his wish to have
a colonoscopy, and he returned for annual visits. However, he didn't follow through
on his intuition. Is this a gender issue? The research says yes.*

According to a survey conducted by Lou Harris and Associates for the Commonwealth Fund, a private foundation in New York, 25 percent of the men polled had not seen a doctor in the last year, compared with just 8 percent of the women, and 30 percent of the men had no regular doctor, compared with only 20 percent of the women.

Part of the reason is sociological. While women are encouraged to listen to their feelings and factor intuition into their decisions, men are raised to "tough it out" and "handle" things. They tend to suppress the inner voice in favor of cold logic, collective experience, and proven formula. For many, a trip to the doctor is an admission of weakness.

The tragic irony, of course, is that Lou did not fit this stereotype. He had a primary care physician and was diligent about his annual visits. Unfortunately, his doctor was afflicted with a not uncommon variant of this machismo: those who make it clear they do not like to be second-guessed.

TREATMENTS AND TRIALS

The traditional treatment for Lou's cancer, according to National Cancer Institute and American Cancer Society guidelines, is surgery followed by radiation and chemotherapy. However, some Internet sources indicate that the trend is toward preoperative chemo and radiation, which seems to improve outcomes. Lou was treated with chemotherapy and radiation for two months, then had colorectal surgery a month after that.

"I was sixty-one. I was hoping I could keep teaching through all this. But it would have been too difficult. I don't have the strength or the motivation now to get up every day and teach and then try to keep up with my treatments. It's just too time-consuming and debilitating. But I try to stay active, because there's always hope for something coming down the pike.

"In fact, I was lucky. The chemotherapies they used at first didn't help, and I was getting worse. I flunked 5FU (Fluoracil) and CPT11 (Camptosar), but almost by accident my wife and I learned about some clinical trials that were having some success. There was nothing published, but we had left the door open for family and friends to notify us if they came across anything that might help my situation. One night an e-mail came through from a good friend giving us the name of a research nurse to call about an ongoing trial, using Oxaliplatin, at the Comprehensive Cancer Center at Roswell Park in Buffalo, New York. She gave us the name of the program director: Dr. Cynthia Gail Liechman.

"Other leads came in as well. We followed them up, talking to secretaries who knew somebody who knew somebody who worked there. We called around and finally got the information. We

The American Cancer Society estimates that 95,000 new cases of colon cancer and 35,000 cases of rectal cancer are diagnosed annually in the United States. An estimated 47,900 people with colon cancer and 8,700 with rectal cancer die from the diseases each year. These cancers are the third most common of all cancers, as well as the third most frequent cause of cancer death in both men and women.

had to do this entirely on our own, and mostly outside the system. The chemotherapy that bought some additional months of tumor shrinkage and relief was Oxaliplatin/5FU/Leucovorin."

In medical research, a clinical trial is a study conducted with patients, usually to evaluate a new treatment. It may be conducted by the National Cancer Institute, a pharmaceutical company, or a medical center. Each study is designed to answer scientific questions and to find new and better ways to help patients. Not everyone is eligible. Each study requires patients with certain types and stages of cancer and certain health standards. For Lou, even the possibility of being included in a clinical trial began to transform his fatigue and despair into determination and hope.

"I tried to get into these clinical trials but was told there was a two-month waiting period. The way my oncologist was talking, I didn't think I had very much time. I made an appointment, and I was going to show up and beg them to let me in because everything else had failed. I had called the day before, and they told me, 'Gee, we're way backed up and we've got all these applicants.'

"Later that day I was talking with someone in my support group. I told him I was going to throw myself on the mercy of these people. He said, 'This may be an opportune time.' It turns out he had a friend who had just dropped out of the same trials. So when I arrived, I talked to the director. She said, 'We just had to drop somebody.' Then she sat there for a minute, and maybe it was the sight of my face that got to her, because she said, 'Well, how would you like to join our program?'

"Of course, we didn't know if it would work. We had to go through a nine-week cycle and then an MRI to find out, but in fact it was doing some good. It reduced the size of some my tumors, and one tumor was completely eliminated. I felt very fortunate.

"And I'm glad I was persistent. We could easily have missed it. The medical system is not set up to help you find out everything that is out there. You have to be an activist. I'm not sure the doctors even have this information. In fact, in a lot of cases I'm sure they don't. There is only so much information out there. Medical practices, in many cases, are being run like a business, not like a profession.

"I'm primarily concerned now with surviving as long as I can, of course, but there's a larger issue. A small but significant number of doctors treat these things so cavalierly that it's a crime, and somebody has to bring this to the public's attention. Fortunately, most doctors are not like this. They live up to their professional commitment and put the patient's welfare first.

"This doctor, the one who put me behind the eight-ball, was a professional. I trusted him and relied on his judgment. And he really let me down. He will end up killing me because he wasn't following the guidelines."

DISCOVERED MOMENTS

The pain of learning the medical system's shortcomings firsthand is balanced by Lou's discovery of a world he had been missing. "When you know the end is near, life gets sweeter. Earlier today I was sitting out in the sun in my backyard, and the sky was so blue, and I thought, Man, I don't want to miss this. I'm sure I had looked at the sky a thousand times before, but I never saw the same depth of blueness, never felt the sun as keenly, and it was warm and comfortable and enjoyable. And I knew I didn't want to give it all up.

"I've got grandchildren, I've got a family, and I want to spend more time with them. I want to extend my life as long as possible. I'm hoping something will come along — vaccination, monoclonal antibodies, herbal remedies, whatever — and just keep me going.

"A lot of things I thought I couldn't live without have really become unimportant. Things I took for granted,

"I'm sure I had looked at the sky a thousand times before, but I never saw the same depth of blueness and I never felt the sun as keenly."

even just feeling good enough to take a three-mile walk, which I try whenever I can, have become a lot more important and a lot more satisfying. A side effect of the radiation therapy is that I have to get up five or six times a night to urinate. But last night I only got up twice. It was a wonderful night. I woke up this morning feeling good, feeling refreshed. It's sort of ridiculous, but that's something I used to take for granted, and now it's a wonderful thing.

"One thing that's changed is how deeply I feel things. The Erie canal runs pretty close to my house. I've always enjoyed walking along the canal banks. It's very peaceful — no traffic, plenty of wildlife. Before, I might see something interesting, but I wouldn't feel it the same way I feel it now. It can be a very moving experience.

"A lot of my sense of taste has disappeared, but occasionally I'll get a meal that I can eat that is really tasty and enjoyable. Eating used to be just automatic. It was just fuel to keep the furnace going so I could go out and write another article or do another consulting job or bank some more money.

"My world was my research and my writing, my teaching. I was a typical workaholic. I thought that work was the be-all and end-all of everything. All of a sudden I realize that other things, relationships and such, are much more important and satisfying.

Common signs and symptoms of colorectal cancer:

- *Change in bowel habits*
- *Diarrhea, constipation, or a feeling that the bowel does not empty completely*
- *Blood (either bright red or very dark) in the stool*
- *Stools that are narrower than usual*
- *General abdominal discomfort (frequent gas pains, bloating, fullness, and/ or cramps)*
- *Weight loss with no known reason*
- *Constant tiredness*
- *Vomiting*

These symptoms may be caused by colorectal cancer or by other conditions. It is important to check with a doctor. Cancer screening guidelines recommend that at age 50, both men and women should follow one of three screening options:

- *Yearly fecal occult blood test plus flexible sigmoidoscopy every 5 years, or*
- *Colonoscopy every 10 years, or*
- *Double contrast barium enema every 5–10 years.*

"This sounds a bit insane, but in a way it was a good thing to have happen. It brought my wife and me closer together; we had been going down separate career paths. And my children and I are a lot closer now. They see what it takes to face pain every day, and it gives me an opportunity, I suppose, to be a little braver than I thought I was."

JOY AND FEAR

"There's a sad sweetness to the whole experience. I'm sort of happy it happened, because it opened my eyes, but at the same time I feel the pain and I don't want to let go. If somebody said, 'We can cure you, but you'll have to give up what you've learned by going through this experience,' of course I would take the cure, but I wouldn't want to give up what I've learned. It's a lesson I don't think I would have learned any other way. Somehow it hooked my mind to my heart, and I began to feel the things that I knew were there intellectually, but I never really got the beauty of the meaning or the depth out of it. And I've heard other people say this — that they felt things so much more keenly as a result of having cancer.

"I wouldn't want to give up what I've learned. Somehow it hooked my mind to my heart."

"I would take the cure, even if I had to give up the learning. But I wouldn't give up the pain. I would suffer the pain I went through to learn the lesson. There was a lot of pain. My operation didn't go well, and there were a lot of complications. I spent nearly nine months in pain, much of it in bed, incapacitated. But I've pushed the pain out of my mind. I hardly think about it anymore.

"But there's also the fear. I wake up every morning, and I have to admit, sometimes it really grabs me. Especially when things are going badly and nothing is working. I'll get that knot in my stomach and I'll think, is this the last time I'll see spring? Is this my last autumn? Is this my last trip to our summer cottage? It's hard to let go of these things, especially when you discover how wonderful they are and realize that any minute they could be taken from you.

"A friend of mine, an older gentleman I used to walk the canal banks with and had known a long time, died of liver cancer. He was visiting down in Florida, and all of a sudden started feeling sick. He just barely got back here, and within a couple of weeks he was dead. It could have been even quicker, like the heart attack my father had, where you have no chance to learn this appreciation for the ordinary things in life, this hypersensitivity to beauty.

"So I've got this consolation — that I've had more time to appreciate these things than a lot of people have had or could have. Whatever time I have left is not a small thing to me. I do appreciate it.

"If someone were to ask me to sum up what I've learned in the form of advice, I would say, 'Appreciate the beauty of the moment.' But I don't think someone who hasn't looked death in the eye can really understand what that means."

When we don't have to think about our health all day, every day, week in and week out, we experience life as a walking tour across a foggy landscape. We know there's an amazing world out there, but it's somewhere beyond the fog, just out of sight, and there are things close up that we need to pay attention to — rocks that we don't want to trip over, fountains that we need to stop and drink from on our way home.

We look around carelessly and think, Someday I'm going to walk out in that direction and see what's over there. It's probably a grand view, but I've got things to do today. Tomorrow will be fine.

Then, one day, walking along as usual, paying attention to nothing in particular, wrapped in our everyday concerns, we suddenly find ourselves at the edge of an abyss. It's a very scary place to be, because although we have known most of our lives that there was an abyss somewhere ahead, we had no idea we were just a few steps away from it. And suddenly we're looking down and down, and there's no bottom anywhere in sight.

It has a way of raising the hair on the back of our neck — and clearing the fog.

We begin to back away from the edge. That way — there's a path over there. It's rocky and it looks painful, but it goes on a ways and it doesn't drop over the edge — not right away, at least. Let's go that way for a while.

Soon our feet are bleeding, and we're tired and feeling sick, but at least the path keeps going.

After a bit, we begin to get used to the razor-sharp stones and the impossibly steep pitches; our feet toughen up, and we breathe a little easier. And we start to look around. The fog has mostly cleared, and we can see many paths that we missed in the fog, and lots of people wandering along them.

Way off on the horizon are ranges of magical mountains, shimmering like a mirage, inviting us to come and visit.

In the middle distance are glorious fields of tall grass waving in the wind, and herds of creatures we have read about but never dared to believe were real.

But stop! Brushing our ankles are the most exquisitely colored and delicately shaped flowers we have ever seen. Were they there before? Why have we never noticed them?

And we realize that it is not the fog that has lifted; there was never any fog, after all. It is our spirits, our minds, that have lifted, and the scales have dropped from our eyes. We can see, for the first time, what was there all along.

And it is beautiful.

4

The Voice of Empowerment

As a Health Care Professional and Public Speaker, Fern Carness has a mission to remind people of the importance of medical self-responsibility. Twenty years ago, her topic would have been cardiac recovery; today, it is empowerment, especially for women who feel at the mercy of an often gender-biased medical community. Don't just watch out for obvious symptoms of disease, she tells her audiences, or accept as received wisdom the advice of medical practitioners. Pay close attention to your inner voice, the one that whispers subtle warnings now and then or nags constantly at the back of your mind, telling you that something is out of whack. Keep your eyes open, she says — and above all, "Be your own first opinion."

Answering questions from her audience, Fern is steady and professional, focusing her attention and expertise on each questioner's concerns. Alone with me, she is less guarded. She tells me her own story of discovery, denial, and a determination to take back control of her own life.

"Keep your eyes open, and above all, be your own first opinion."

"Every year in May since I turned thirty-five, I've had a mammogram on my birthday. Even though I was below the recommended age, I had fairly cystic, lumpy breasts, so I thought it was just a good thing to do. I'm a nurse, and I've worked in radiology in a lot of hospitals.

"I'd had a mammogram two years in a row at the same place. The second year I went, the technician who did the mammogram was very inexperienced, and I had an omen. I remember thinking at the time, *Mark this moment.* But when I got the results, there was no problem.

"The year after that, I got a mammogram at a health fair I had put together for a client. Again, no problem. But there was a problem with the mammograms that day, and we had to write a couple of letters apologizing to two women whose mammograms got mixed up. This made a little alarm go off in my mind that something might be wrong.

"Two and a half months later, in July, I popped into the shower one morning, and as my hand ran across my breast, just doing the regular soapy dopey, I hit a stone in my breast the size of golf ball and just as hard, dimpled and absolutely not human, and the minute my hand touched it, my brain said, 'This is cancer.'

"I'd practiced the self-exam regularly, but I did have very lumpy breasts, so it could have been difficult to differentiate. But I thought, How could this lump not have been there yesterday, and here it is today, the size of a damn tangerine?

"The fact is," said Fern, "it's very common. Breast cancer is very insidious. It infiltrates and thickens, and you may not notice the gradual thickening until it reaches a sort of critical mass and causes an inflammation around it, and then you can suddenly feel the lump. It's more the reaction of the tissue around the cancer that causes the lump, rather than the cancer itself."

THE GOOD LIFE, INTERRUPTED

Fern and her husband are a modern American success-story family, accustomed to controlling their lives and enjoying their good health and material success. And as a health-promotion professional, Fern practices what she preaches. For virtually her entire adult life, she has modeled proper nutrition, regular exercise, stress management, abstinence from tobacco, and moderate use of alcohol. But cancer, like many other of life's rude interruptions, does not discriminate; it's an equal-opportunity aggressor, and it plays by its own rules.

"I was forty-one years old. I owned a worksite wellness company that serviced all of California, good annual gross revenue, with ten full-time employees and a hundred part-timers, and I'm queen of wellness for Southern California — national speaker, size four, tan, petite, married to a man who has an international musical instrument manufacturing and distribution business. We're bringing in a chunk of money, we have two lovely sons in private schools, we live in Southern California, swimming pool, movie stars, the whole deal.

"And suddenly, there it was. A lump.

"So, as I felt this, a wave of icy terror went through me. I knew it was cancer. Not because I'm a nurse and not because I'm a health educator — I just knew it as a woman, that this was a piece of nonhuman stuff inside my body.

"I stepped out of the shower, and the phone was ringing. It was my office secretary trying to tell me that we forgot a power cord on a health-fair site and somebody would have to run it out to the team, and then my pager went off and it was the people on the health-fair site telling me they didn't have their power cord, and one of my kids needed lunch money and the other one needed car keys, and I remembered my husband said something about six Japanese dignitaries coming to dinner that night and I wondered if the housekeeper had everything under control, and so I just grabbed the blow dryer and went on with my entire day and never gave what happened in the shower another thought.

"I can't really believe it when I look back on it. How did I step out of that shower, knowing I had cancer, and walk right back into my life and never give it a second thought?

"I didn't think about it again until later that night, after the Japanese guys had left. My husband and I were making love, and suddenly it was lights on, romance off. He said, 'What in the world is that?' I said, 'Oh, yeah, I forgot about that. I was going to call my doctor.' And he's like, 'What do you mean, you forgot?' It was terrible. He could tell, and he was terrified because it felt so horrible and so big.

"The next morning I went to my OB/GYN's office at nine,

Fern refers to the lump as not being "human." Of course the tissue is human, but the horror of its discovery is so shocking and disruptive and fearful that a common response is detachment and denial. An invasion has occurred, and the alien is so frightening that the little kid inside wants to pull the blanket over her head, cover her ears, and keep very, very still until the monster goes away.

without an appointment, just walked in and said I needed to see him right away. Now, this is the doctor who's been seeing me since I was eighteen, delivered both of my children, was my proctor in nursing school, a really nice guy. He loved me. So they sent me right in. He checked the lump and said, 'You know, it's probably a cyst. You have a lot of fibroids. It's probably no big deal. Why don't we give it one or two menstrual cycles?'

"So I left there feeling relieved for the moment, but then I kept having this gnawing feeling that he was wrong. And I started thinking about how in the last few weeks I had had a cold, and the flu, and a sinus infection, and an earache, and how unusual that was because I'm never sick. And then I thought, well, if my body's busy fighting off a big old cancer it probably doesn't have any energy left for keeping the common cold at bay. And I became very upset and depressed."

THE RELUCTANT DOCTOR

"I went back the next morning without an appointment. This time it took them a couple of hours to squeeze me in, and as I waited in the office, I started sobbing. I tried to call my husband, but it was one of those nightmares where you try to dial a number, and you lose track, and then you hang up and try again, but it's busy, and you try again, but you get 'The number you dialed is not a working number.'

Part of what saved Fern's life was her focus. Once she realized something was indeed wrong, she set out to get more information. Her doctor may have felt that it was nothing to be too concerned with, but her senses told her differently. No matter how devastating the truth might be, she had to know — and know immediately.

"By the time the doctor came in to examine me, I was freaking out. He said, 'Fern, you're hysterical. I'm going to medicate you and get hold of your husband and have somebody pick you up.' I said, 'I probably am hysterical and probably should be medicated, but you need to put a needle in this, and you need to do it right now, because I'm not leaving here until you do.'

"He said, 'First of all, I'm not a surgeon. We need a breast guy to do it. And it's a holiday weekend.' And I said, 'You know what, Gordon, it doesn't matter. I'm not leaving this fucking office until somebody takes a look at this with a needle. If you can't do it, give me the stuff and I'll do it myself, because I know this is malignant.'"

Fern says that, in retrospect, her doctor's biggest problem may have been denial. He was a dear friend, and although he was a doctor and should have known better, he simply didn't want to think his friend might have cancer. "He cared so much he couldn't see it." Perhaps more to the point, he cared so much he didn't want to see it. At that point, however, Fern had sped through denial and was looking for quick, decisive action.

"So the long and short of it — they called in a surgeon. I went upstairs to get a biopsy. Now, I'm a nurse, so when he popped the needle in there to aspirate, and he hit solid granite, I knew we were in trouble. He's saying, 'Well, we'll send this off to pathology, and we'll give you a call Monday morning and let you know the good news,' and I'm thinking, Liar, liar, liar!

"Then I went downstairs to get another mammogram — post-biopsy, to compare with the one I got before the biopsy. I was wearing this peach sundress, which I haven't been able to wear since — it was a cute little skimpy braless thing. By now I was so upset that I couldn't breathe, couldn't speak, and I got the written order for the

Most people are very passive when it comes to dealing with their physicians, often responding with blank stares, silent nodding, and questions that never reach the tongue. The doctor is perceived as a kind of god who must be blindly obeyed, and the patient is embarrassed or concerned about looking stupid. The result is that the doctor fights the battle alone — without the benefit of patient observation and intuition. Had Fern listened to her primary care physician's recommendation to wait two more menstrual cycles, or had she believed the initial interpretation of her mammogram, she would certainly have faced metastatic cancer. It was her courage to explore, speak, and be heard that saved her life.

mammogram mixed up with my parking stub and accidentally dropped them both on the receptionist's desk. Without looking up, she said, 'We don't validate.' I stood there with my face all swollen and tears running down. I could have killed her.

"We did the mammogram, and the radiologist came in and said, 'Well, Mrs. Carness, I don't know why you're so hysterical, because your mammogram looks fine.' I made him put his hand on my lump, and I said to him, 'Do you need X-ray vision to see this?' He freaked out, because he didn't see it on my X-ray. A solid, six-centimeter, stage three, malignant tumor, and he couldn't see it.

"This scares me when I teach other women about mammograms and self-examination, because, like many women, I have very dense breasts, which are the kind you want if you're looking for *Baywatch* opportunities, but they make it hard to see tumors in a mammogram.

"He went over the mammograms again, and he was very nervous. He started seeing stuff where he didn't see anything before, maybe this or maybe that, and by the time I walked out of there we were both totally confused.

"The weekend was tense. My husband tried to cheer me up. He said, 'Wait till Monday. Don't worry until you have to.' But it was still a long, hard weekend for me."

WAITING FOR THE OTHER SHOE

Going back to work was not easy, says Fern. "I was supposed to work in the cardiac catheter lab Monday morning, but I had my own business to run and had decided not to go in. However, one of the nurses called at 5:00 A.M. and said they had three cardiac emergencies and asked me to come in. I said I couldn't, I was waiting for some biopsy results. Like a typical nurse, she said, 'You can wait for the results while you're working.'

"So I went to work, and after a while my pager went off. It was the phone number of the surgeon. I called him back, and he said, 'Why don't you come on down, and we'd like to give you a biopsy report, and by the way, could you bring a family member and all of your mammograms?'

"I knew what this meant. I said to myself, Do they treat regular people this stupidly? I was terrified, but as a health educator, I was angry.

"So my husband came and we went to the surgeon's office. I was still in scrubs. I even had the blue booties over my sneakers. The surgeon told us it was malignant and recommended a modified radical mastectomy. Then he stopped speaking to me. He looked at my husband and said, 'We'll have a plastic surgeon on standby. She'll go to sleep with two breasts and she'll wake up with two breasts. You'll never even know she had cancer.' He said this to my husband as if I were no longer in the room.

"My husband said nothing. He didn't breathe. We'd been married twenty-two years, and he knew better. It was as if I had asked, 'Do I look fat in these jeans?'

"I said to the doctor, 'Excuse me, but did anybody ask if I want to be reconstructed? You just told me I have cancer. I don't know exactly what that means to my life. I don't know whether I'm going to live or die, and you want to know if I want to have nice tits?' I said, 'I don't know that I want to be reconstructed, and I need to think about it.'

"And the doctor said, 'Now, Fern, look how cute and sexy you are, and you're young. Don't you want to be a woman?'

"I don't think he meant to hurt me. I think the man was genuinely trying to be helpful. Which was the saddest part of it.

Put yourself in Fern's shoes for a moment. You are an experienced nurse and health promotion specialist, dedicated to the principles of medical self-responsibility. Following those principles, you have discovered a tumor in your breast. In spite of well-intentioned roadblocks, you plow your way through the health care system, pleading for a comprehensive examination. You endure a needle biopsy and wait in agonized suspense while the results are analyzed. The physician tells you that you have malignant cancer and your breast will have to come off. Then he turns to your husband and tells him not to worry because when you go to sleep they will build you a new breast and he won't be able to tell you had cancer. Now — how do you feel?

"He then said, 'Well, if you like, you can get a second opinion.' And that's when I got angry.

"I said, 'Dr. Bernstein, you *are* the second opinion. *My* opinion was the first. I count here.'

"In the empowerment talks I now present to breast cancer patients, I use this line: 'Be your own first opinion.' I tell them, 'You have to know your body.'"

MORE OPINIONS

Fern had two days to prepare for the operation and decide whether or not to undergo reconstruction. She called a cancer hotline and was told she would be mailed some information — which would arrive too late to help. The Internet was embryonic, and she didn't have the time or emotional strength to dig through her community library's limited resources.

"I had one son in college, another in high school, and I was forty-one. I was just trying to get things in order. My sister was planning on coming down to help. Somebody brought over *Dr. Susan Love's Breast Book*, but I wouldn't even look at it because I thought it was going to tell me I was going to die.

"So I did what every good Jewish-American princess does when she's stressed out. I went to the mall, and I spent an entire day just walking up and down the mall, buying nothing. I had nothing to buy. I just walked up and down, trying to sort it out in my mind and get things organized.

"I wanted to find out whether reconstruction would make it harder to monitor for reoccurrence. I called five oncologists. The first four, I couldn't get past the nurse because I wasn't referred by another doctor. The fifth nurse

Fortunately, today there are many credible and reliable Internet sources affiliated with the National Cancer Institute and the American Cancer Society that can help cancer patients find research information as they ponder critical treatment decisions. But Fern had to rely on limited printed material and her personal determination to seek out skilled professional support.

said, 'Dr. Charles would tell you, but he's on vacation and won't be back until Monday.' This was Wednesday; I was having surgery on Thursday. But she called back an hour later and gave me the number of the doctor's brother, another physician. "I called the brother and asked him my question. He was very nice. He told me he understood my dilemma. 'But I really can't advise you,' he said. 'I've never seen you. I haven't met you. I haven't seen your clinical situation. I just don't know what to say.'

"I said, 'Okay, I understand that. But I'm a cardiovascular nurse specialist, and you sound to me like a short, balding, overweight, forty-five-year old man, and let me tell you that if you get chest pain, and you're not sure whether you want an angioplasty or a PTCA or TPA or if you think you should just jump in and have a heart transplant, you give me a call. Save my number, and I'll at least give you my ballpark opinion.'

"He said, 'Don't get reconstructed.'

"I said, 'Thank you, sir,' and hung up.

"Now, look what I had to go through to get a few answers. And I'm in the medical profession. Most people wouldn't have the chutzpah. They wouldn't even know where to start.

"I want to make one point. I decided not to get a same-sitting reconstruction. Many women are encouraged to do it, not only for the beauty of having two breasts, but also because a managed care company will be more likely to pay for it because it's only one surgery. But women are ill-prepared to make that decision under these circumstances, and you can reserve the right to be reconstructed any time you want, even ten years later. There's a federal law, the Women's and Children's Cancer Act, that says if you have the insurance, they must pay for it, whenever it happens."

UNDER THE KNIFE

Fern had a regular mastectomy and lymph node dissection, then went into six months of chemotherapy. One lymph node had cancer cells, but her bones were clear. Her prognosis was good. But she had crippling doubts.

"I thought for sure, with my diagnosis, that I would go through chemo but die anyway. I was a cardiovascular nurse, and I didn't know much about cancer. I just thought everybody who got cancer died.

"So the first thing I had to do was recognize how angry I was — and I was very angry. I thought it was unfair, and I didn't think that I had any part in the manifestation of this cancer. I didn't understand the things I now understand about the mind-body connection.

"I began to learn a lot from people like Candace Pert and Louise Hay and Bernie Segal and others about controlling my outcome. I opened my head and heart to a more holistic approach — mind, body, and spirit. Prayer. Guided imagery. Friendship. I could, in Bernie Segal's words, 'become an exceptional cancer patient.' I could do a better job of survival by putting my mind to it. But that frightened me too, because if I could be held accountable for improving my outcome, couldn't I also be held responsible for building the cancer in the first place? Could I accept that responsibility?"

Fern's doubt, anger, and confusion are typical. A diagnosis of cancer often brings out the lawyer in those who receive it. Somebody must have done something wrong; the doctor messed up; I messed up. Many assume that something, no matter how remote the possibility, will go wrong, and that they must be prepared for it. Despite her favorable prognosis, Fern's lack of cancer knowledge, combined with her anger, made it difficult for her to digest all the information she was getting and to be objective.

Fern elected not to accept the guilt but to pour all her energy into healing. "I decided to take responsibility for the recovery but not the cancer." She knew, and frequently passed along the information to others, that except for lung cancer and smoking there is little connection between lifestyle and cancer. The risk is higher with certain factors, such as diet, alcohol consumption, and stress, but the link is neither direct nor uniform. And genetics, which no one can choose, plays a strong role — so it's always a good idea to be familiar with your family's medical history.

FINDING THE GIFTS

Like others who have faced down the looming possibility of death, Fern has discovered the dual nature of such threats. The positive aspects are often seen as benefits — gifts — that might never have been realized without the threat of an imminent demise.

"Cancer gave me a wonderful gift. People used to tell me this early on: 'Oh, this happened for a reason. You'll see. Cancer can be a blessing in disguise.' I would say, 'I don't need any more gifts, thank you. I was doing just fine.' But in fact I did get some wonderful gifts.

"One of these gifts was the ability to be selfish. Well, not really selfish, but self-nurturing. It gave me the ability to say no. I started evaluating the hundreds of people in my life. Most of them were energy takers, not energy givers, and I really didn't enjoy many of them. They weren't my friends; they were my employees or acquaintances or colleagues, but I had mistaken them for friends. So I realized I didn't have the quality of friendships that I thought I had, and that I didn't have to be in a relationship if I didn't want to be. Like, 'If I'm going to die, are you the person I want to spend my last day with?' And 'Even if I'm not going to die, do I want to waste a day with you?' So the gift is that now I have wonderfully deep friendships with people, better than any I had before."

As if the pain and physical discomfort were not enough to deal with, cancer in the family often brings other, long-standing problems to the surface. Shaky relationships deteriorate; overstrained finances

We are just beginning to understand some of the many environmental factors that contribute to the risk of cancer. Certainly, you should exercise, not smoke, drink only in moderation or not at all, and limit your dietary fat — but this is no guarantee against cancer. The best course is to pay attention to your body, react quickly when you sense something wrong, and get professional intervention at the earliest sign of disease. Leave the guilt behind; concentrate on being as healthy as you can.

crumble; children on the emotional edge lose their balance. But the cancer that precipitates these crises can also focus one's attention on resolving them.

"I'm a little more self-centered about my time now," says Fern. "I was terrified about dying before my children were ready. My younger son got heavily involved in drugs during my chemo time, and we had a lot of family work to do to save his life. Once we were sure we had him in a place where he would live, the question was, could we help him turn his own life around? And I'm proud to say that he graduated from the University of Oregon last December, and he seems to be getting in line to be a productive, wonderful guy and maybe going to law school."

When you experience a serious health crisis like cancer, for a time all you think about is the possibility of dying. You cry, shake your fist, become philosophical, tend to practical matters, perform acts of contrition, and explore visions of the next world. Then, when good medicine and your better nature begin to turn you once again toward living, you start to focus on what kind of life will you lead. You do so knowing one thing for certain — it will not be the same as it was before you were diagnosed. You are forever changed. You can proudly wear the mantle of "cancer survivor," or you can move to the next level as a "cancer thriver." People in this latter group are buoyed by their cancer experience and begin to develop a wonderful sense of metaphysical arrogance. They resolve to take hold of their life and shape their destiny. Fern is one of thousands of members of this thriver club. She has shaped her destiny with the most powerful force of all — love.

KNOWING WHAT MATTERS

"I learned that the only thing that matters is love. I told myself, Okay, if I'm going to die, what's this been about? What do I take away from this life, and what do I leave behind? The only thing that kept coming back was love — love for my children, my husband, my sister. Love for my profession — I love caring for patients. I decided I should stay on this planet a little bit longer; I have more to contribute.

"I made a list of ten things I wouldn't get to do if I died while I was going through this stuff. Things like, I hadn't been to the Grand Canyon. I had never left the country, unless you count going to Club Med, which I don't count. I had never learned to whistle really loud, like my sister, with two fingers in my mouth.

"And then I tried to make a list of regrets, but the only regret I could come up with was that I had not danced enough. I love to dance, but my husband doesn't. So for about three years after my diagnosis, I went dancing without my husband every Wednesday night, and I had a blast. I went to this little honky-tonk where everybody knew I was married and was just there to dance, just for the joy of moving my body to music."

Fern takes on life wearing her best dancing shoes and a take-no-prisoners attitude. Decades from now, the words of Dylan Thomas will ring loud and clear for her:

> Do not go gentle into that good night,
> Old age should burn and rave at close of day;
> Rage, rage against the dying of the light.

Just as Fern's six-centimeter tumor should not have required X-ray vision to detect, we often ignore or deny problems that threaten to grow quickly beyond our ability to control them. We feel them, but we choose not to see them. What saved Fern was paying attention to a gut feeling that all was not right with her body, regardless of what others were telling her. Beyond her training as a nurse, she knew that something was wrong, and she kept making noise until she got the attention she needed.

After careful consideration of personal psychosocial factors and the advice of a physician, Fern chose to forgo immediate reconstructive surgery so that, if the cancer came back, she would be able to detect the tumor at the earliest possible stage. Her decision was neither "correct" nor "incorrect." It was simply the right decision for her — not necessarily for every woman. In Fern's opinion (the first opinion), it boiled down to choosing clarity over cosmetics.

In our own lives, it is tempting to see only what we want to see. We pretend that all is well, hoping that time will heal everything. Warning signs flash at us, screaming for attention, while we look away, afraid to confront the issue head-on. What if I fail? What if I make the wrong decision? What if there really is something seriously wrong? Just as Fern's shower discovery was pushed to the back of her mind by thoughts of her dinner party and her work, we all get so caught up in the routine of living that we sometimes miss or ignore serious issues — or issues that may become serious if we don't take care of them early.

It was a long time before Fern could derive value from her trip to the edge. She experienced anger, fear, resentment, and a healthy dose of "Why me?" Having spent her career as a health professional, she didn't feel she needed further reminders of the importance of medical self-responsibility. However, as months passed, she began to discover the gifts of cancer. Time became more precious, friendships were more valued, and she learned to laugh at herself and her situation. She has discovered a new career as an author and national speaker, and now uses her experience to help others.

How have you responded to crisis and tragedy in your life? How will you in the future? Take a page from Fern's life: try a little chutzpah.

5

The Voice of Engagement

HIS 1973 DRIVER'S LICENSE BIRTHDATE NOTWITHSTANDING, Matthew Cummins seems wise beyond his years. He is an engineer by training and inclination, a logical man, but he keeps an artist's eye for the subtleties and imponderables of life. Some of this comes from his experience, some from his role models.

"The people I look up to, the ones I choose as mentors, are people who are fully engaged in their work, their art, their hobbies," says Matthew. "In life. In their careers. In religion, some of them. They're active; they're engaged. They have passion. They celebrate life.

"I want my life to be a work of art. But I've been trained as an engineer to be analytical, so I've always found a contradiction there. As a perfectionist, I find it hard to think of my life as a work of art. I get frustrated. I put too much pressure on myself. I'm never as good at appreciating life as I'd like to be. Sometimes I find myself trying too hard to make it something special."

POET AND PRAGMATIST

"I've always loved solving things, which is why I became an engineer. In high school, I was into both academics and athletics, but my identity was shaped mostly by my grade point average and being valedictorian. I was drawn to intellectual pursuits.

"In my part of the Midwest — I grew up in Grand Rapids, Michigan — if you were smart, if you applied yourself academically, I think it tended to manifest itself in science or math, because there was less exposure to art or world culture. So, naturally, when I entered Stanford I went into mechanical engineering. But I also took some economics

classes, some computer programming, some art. I was not very focused. I was playing, socializing a lot, but my education was going
nowhere fast. And in a place like Stanford, that's a real waste of an
opportunity.

"But Stanford has this neat policy that lets you step out for as
long as you need and then just show up again when you're ready to
go back to school. So I decided to take a year off. My parents thought
I was making a mistake, but I needed it. I had been in a pretty tense
academic and work environment for a long time.

"First thing I did, I biked across the country from Seattle to Washington, D.C. It was for a fund-raising event called Bike Aid, but I was
doing it purely for escape. After that I took odd jobs, worked for my
father for a few months, then got into an engineering internship.

"After a year, I was ready to go back to school and apply myself.
What I was really interested in, I decided, was materials. This was a
really exciting field of engineering. Twenty or thirty years ago, materials meant metallurgy, but now it's metals, ceramics, plastics, and
silicones — everything from better tennis rackets to microchips."

A Decision Overridden

Matthew settled into his studies and set his sights on a career that
seemed assured. Stanford is a place where school and life can be
richly enjoyed — the academic stimulation of a top-ranked school,
the siren song of Northern California's seacoast, mountains, red-
woods, sports, and culture. These are the things a college student
who has earned such a promising opportunity expects to enjoy.

The last thing he expects is a heart attack. "At the end of the spring
quarter, during final exam week, I woke up in the middle of the
night with intense chest pains and a numb left arm. My reaction was,
I have an exam in a few hours, I don't have time to have a heart
attack. Shows you how out of whack a Stanford student's priorities
can get.

"I sat still and took long breaths until I could control the pain a
little. After a while I went back to sleep. I woke up in the morning
and took the exam. The next night, the pain came back.

"So I went to the emergency room, and they checked me over and said it was probably stress because of exam week, or maybe an infection. They gave me some antibiotics. "That night the pain was even worse. I went back and they gave me a shot to relax my muscles. They checked me over again and everything looked good. But then a sharp-eyed radiologist reviewed my X-rays and noticed that my sternum looked a little wider than normal. So they did some CT scans.

"And that's when they found the tumor in my chest. A big one. The size of a Rubik's Cube, right behind my sternum.

"Now, the interesting aspect of this is that they hadn't been able to contact me for a few days, and in the meantime I had been taking the antibiotics and the pain had completely cleared up. So the pain may not have been caused by the tumor. It may have been just a stroke of luck that got me checked out."

FATE

Matthew is an engineer, and as he points out, engineers tend to be linear thinkers who believe in the logic of cause and effect. However, Matthew the Poet had often felt caught in the grip of something bigger than himself, something he didn't quite understand. Of his ten closest college friends, the ones he had stayed in touch with, three had been diagnosed with cancer. Two of them had Hodgkin's lymphoma, the same disease Matthew's doctors had found in him. This was statistically highly unlikely, since only 7,000 cases a year are diagnosed.

Other than a possible elevated risk associated with having once contracted

Some cancer signs are more obvious than others. A bloody discharge from a nipple, a sore that won't heal, coughing up blood, and a mole that has changed dramatically are all pretty clear messages that cancer is a possibility. However, as in Matthew's situation, cancer can also disguise itself as something else or hide until it has had time to grow into a monster. In those cases it takes a patient smart enough to seek help, a conscientious caregiver, and perhaps a good measure of luck.

mononucleosis, Hodgkin's appears to strike indiscriminately. It is probably just coincidence that Matthew's Uncle Mike was diagnosed with the same disease years earlier, before Matthew left Grand Rapids. Coincidence — but perhaps strangely prophetic.

Matthew had been in his Uncle Mike's hospital room the night he died. "He was so drugged up, he didn't know me. He thought I was his old high school buddy. He was pretty incoherent all night, but at one point he looked at me intently and said, 'Matt, go to the closet and get my shoes, because you and I are going to California.'

"At the time, everybody thought that was a pretty incoherent thing to say. After all, this was a year before I had even applied to Stanford. I didn't remember this until five years later, when I was diagnosed with Hodgkin's — and discovered that the number-one place in the world for research and treatment of Hodgkin's disease is Stanford."

FOCUS

At times during the discovery, diagnosis, and treatment of cancer, the intensity of the experience is so overpowering that the mind, body, and spirit screen out much of the horror of what is happening, both the real and the imagined. Everything is distorted; the patient hears the words, feels the needle sticks, catches his breath between the waves of nausea. The frightened child inside is comforted; he may remember for a while, but he soon forgets the worst of it.

After his diagnosis early that summer, Matthew spent the first two months in chemotherapy, then a month of his fall quarter undergoing radiation treatment. He stayed in school, dealing with the fear, discomfort, and inconvenience by taking a reduced course load — radiation in the morning, classes in the afternoon. "I got the best grades of my whole college career during that quarter," he laughs.

Like many people who are forced to battle cancer, Matthew found himself more focused on life. Once past the shock of the diagnosis, he felt inspired to fight — and not just for his own recovery; he counseled his three friends who had been diagnosed with cancer.

"I told them, 'Keep a journal, because although you're not going to believe me, these things that seem so ominous and feel so intense — like there's no way you could ever forget anything that's happening to you — you get past them and they fade.'"

Matthew reflects, "I have to say, though, that although I've become sort of numb to the whole process, the whole emotion of cancer, some of the details are very, very vivid in my memory. And I'm still working through these things."

LAUGH IT OFF

Matthew handles the seriousness of his situation with a healthy sense of humor. He has quickly learned to appreciate the ironies his life hands him — such as a visit to the sperm bank, an option many young men facing chemotherapy and radiation choose in order to preserve their potential for fatherhood..

Matthew smiles and shakes his head as he remembers the day. "You haven't been through anything until you're a twenty-one-year-old kid sitting in a room with your parents, discussing the possibility of freezing your sperm.

"The nurse comes into the room and, in front of my parents, asks me if I've ejaculated within the last forty-eight hours.

"Even if it had been the day after my wedding night, I probably would have said, 'Oh, no, ma'am!'"

Chemotherapy is designed to kill off aggressive

Some people with Hodgkin's disease have no symptoms at all. Most people with this disease have one or more painless, enlarged lymph nodes that may grow very slowly. But Hodgkin's disease is a very rare cause of lymph node swelling. Especially in children, most lymph node enlargement is due to infection, and the node returns to its normal size within weeks after the infection goes away. Cancers other than Hodgkin's disease can also cause lymph node swelling. If you or your child have lymph nodes over an inch in size, especially if there is no history of a current or recent infection, it is best to have the lymph node examined by a doctor so any disease needing treatment can be found without delay.

cells. However, in addition to attacking the cancer cells, the chemicals also take aim on other fast-growing cells, such as those that produce hair. Some cancer patients go with the "bald-is-beautiful" look; others cover up. Friends don't always know what's up on top.

"A close friend of mine, who had left to study abroad while I was being treated and had lost all my hair, came back a year later. I had by then grown this thick head of hair because I didn't cut it for the first eight months after it grew back. She came up and gave me a big hug and ran her hand through my hair and said, 'God, your hair!' And this look of horror came on her face. 'Wait. Is it real?'

"I woke up early one morning when I had a CAT scan scheduled. I was supposed to drink two big bottles of barium sulfate before going to the hospital. If there's one thing the world needs, it's better-tasting barium sulfate. So I drank the first one — kind of choked it down, I wasn't feeling well that day — and then the second one. Finally I got it all down.

> "Then I realized my appointment
> was the next day."

Scientists have found a few risk factors that may make a person more likely to develop Hodgkin's disease. There seems to be a slightly increased rate of Hodgkin's disease in people who have had infectious mononucleosis ("mono" for short), an infection caused by the Epstein-Barr virus. However, there is no evidence of a previous Epstein-Barr virus infection in half of the patients with Hodgkin's disease, so its role is unclear.

Unlike many other types of cancer, Hodgkin's disease does not seem to be caused by something wrong with a person's genes or diet, or even environmental factors. Certain families have been described with many family members who develop Hodgkin's disease, but this doesn't seem to be caused by a problem with their genes. Even if someone does have one or more risk factors for Hodgkin's disease, it is impossible to know for sure how much that risk factor contributed to causing the cancer.

Since scientists and doctors have not yet found risk factors associated with most cases of Hodgkin's disease, it is not now possible to prevent the disease. Information about suspected risk factors has not yet been translated into practical ways to prevent Hodgkin's disease.

NEW INSIGHTS

Friendships have always been important to Matthew, but when his friends began to join him as new inductees in the cancer club, their shared experience and unspoken understanding deepened the relationships. One of Matthew's friends, a year after treatment, ran in the San Diego Marathon. "She's crazy," he laughs. "But that's part of survival. You get to be a little crazy. The marathon was a fund-raiser for lymphoma, and she asked me if it would be all right if she ran the race for me because of all the help I had given her. I thought that was cool. It reminded me of how much we matter to each other.

"There are two different ways I could react to the fact that my friends are going to keep getting cancer. One way is to be afraid, and pissed off, each time someone gets cancer. The other way is to realize that it's part of life, that good things can come from bad. And this positive reaction seems to be coming more and more to the front. It's given me the ability to take a closer look around me, to rethink some of my conclusions about the way things are. It's given me an appreciation for life. It's made me a much more tolerant person, someone who can empathize more with people.

"I never had the reaction that I commonly read about, the feeling of 'Why is this happening to me?' The 'It's not fair, I hate my God' reaction. You have to be alive in order to have cancer. Dead people don't get cancer.

"Maybe I think that way because of my Uncle Mike. It just makes sense to me. If you honestly celebrate life, then you have to acknowledge that people do get cancer, and that

Matthew celebrates life by accepting death. He appreciates joy by respecting the role of pain; he treasures the fragile gift of health because he acknowledges the existence of disease; he cherishes his friendships because he knows that, without companionship, his tears, laughter, and wonder would find no echo. He understands that to be truly engaged, you must accept life as a continuum that includes joy, sorrow, logic, irony — and most of all, opportunity.

people die. I can understand why people kick and scream and cry and complain, and I wonder if maybe I'm missing something. But I guess I have too much of the engineer in me, the pragmatist, to lament my fate. That wasn't going to help me get through it.

"I wish I could remember where I read it, but there was this quote from a cancer patient, I don't know who: 'I asked my God how much time I had left, and God replied, "Enough to make a difference."' I think that's a good outlook on the future.

"There's an inscription on the wall in Stanford Cathedral that says that if each of us were to take our burdens, our troubles, our sorrows, and wrap them up in a package and throw them all on a common pile, there isn't one among us who, walking up and looking at all the other packages, wouldn't gladly pick up our own again.

"Even though that's a slightly romanticized view of things," adds Matthew, "I do feel strongly that, although I don't know the reason, I'm here for a purpose. Life is a privilege, for as long as I get to be here."

We all set goals, prepare for life as best we can, and map out what we think will be our future; but none of us can expect to follow the map without regard to the twists, turns, washouts, and detours we find on the road stretching before us in the real world. Nor can we imagine that the rougher detours will turn us toward other, more rewarding, destinations than those we envisioned, or at least afford us an opportunity to choose another route.

Young Matthew had the universe in the palm of his hand. He had every reason to expect a successful life as a talented engineer who would make discoveries and change the world. But as the saying goes, "Men plan, God laughs."

Matthew's map has changed. His destination remains the same, but he's on a different road. He is resourceful and adaptable; he will continue to use his engineer's mind and artist's spirit to explore ways around the washouts fate has thrown in his path.

Which leads us to questions each one of us should ask himself or herself: Am I truly engaged in life, or am I just cherry-picking experiences based on a narrow view of my personal universe? Does my world consist of wall-to-wall work and the odd hour

with my immediate family? Do friends, a healthy lifestyle, and my spiritual develop-
ment take a back seat to Monday Night Football*? Am I sacking away money for the*
for a vacation that I won't have time to take? Did I forget to call Bill on his birthday
last week?

Now imagine you are Matthew and ask yourself these questions once again. Are
the answers more poignant? Is time slipping away a little faster? Does the world seem
a little more magical?

6

The Voice of Wisdom

RICKY SNEAFELL, FORTY-THREE, IS A SUCCESSFUL BUSINESSWOMAN, dedicated nurse, and single mom. She recently became president of a growing high-tech company. She has, in recent years, discovered reserves of energy, intellect, interpersonal skills, compassion, and courage. Five years ago, she discovered quite suddenly that she had breast cancer.

Ricky's cancer showed itself suddenly and without any warning. "I came home from work one Friday night, tired from a trip. I took off my work clothes, and as I was undressing, I glanced in the mirror, and my chest looked like a road map. I had all this backed-up vein engorgement and these blue lines, just beautiful-looking, like river tributaries. My skin around the veins was shiny and stretched. I wasn't in pain — I have a high pain tolerance — but my left breast was almost twice the size of my right breast. When I pushed on my breast, I felt a smooth rounded nodule."

Her immediate reaction was typical of many people who encounter something frighteningly amiss in their body: denial. As a nurse, Ricky should have known better, but it struck her as funny. "I thought, You know, even in those Mark Eden bust-enhancement courses, you figure it will work symmetrically."

THE WISDOM OF A CHILD

Ricky trained as a nurse at Columbia University, New York City. She spent part of her class time among walls covered not with anatomy charts but with crayon drawings of rainbows, sunflowers, and balloons. "While I was in training as a clinician," says Ricky, "part of the time I specialized in pediatric oncology. I was quite moved by these young children, who were dealing with death and dying. They never gave up hope, yet they had a deep intuition about what was going on, about the inevitability of death in some cases, and in some respects were more at peace with it than their parents.

"I was incredibly touched by these kids. They would draw pictures of angels, and they would often describe a 'light in the tunnel' that they saw when they went through surgery. They would tell us about angels who spoke to them and said that everything would be fine.

"It made me think there was something beyond the physical and medical side of the world, something spiritual happening beyond what we could explain, that people touched by chronic illness seemed to be able to tap into — perhaps another kind of energy that people were able to reach when their physical energy was running low.

"As a caretaker, I was already aware of the power of human touch. When the children were in pain, I could make them feel better by touching or hugging them. It always brought a smile to their faces.

"So, from these children, I learned that death doesn't have to be something you fear. There was actually a profound peacefulness that came over these kids when they were at the end. It's more of an issue for those left behind. The children who were dying — and this was twenty years ago, when cancer was more like a death sentence — weren't afraid for themselves so much as for their parents and brothers and sisters and how they were going to cope after they had died. Their concern was outside themselves.

"There was another thing. The treatments twenty years ago were so harsh and debilitating

Young children live in an ever-changing world of instinct, wonder, and imagination. Adults see sharp instruments and medical bills but can look ahead to a pain-free future much like their past; the alternative is an inconceivable and unbearable loss. Children live in the present, fully experiencing the joy or pain of the moment, but can easily lose themselves in a magic world of talking dinosaurs and friendly wizards. Thus, to a child, the end of real life can mean an end to the pokes, prods, pain, and nausea and the beginning of dancing with angels in the clouds. This is why children often approach physical death more peacefully than adults.

that after a point many of these children didn't feel they could stand any more. The family wanted to do whatever had to be done to prolong their lives. The children wouldn't say so to their families — they wanted to be strong for their loved ones — but they would tell me quietly, in their own way, when they were ready, that it wasn't what they wanted, or they would draw their desire to be taken by the angels in a picture; they just wanted to rest. But they weren't given any choice. Again and again children would tell me right before they fell asleep, 'No one's asked me what I want.'

"And they were right. So often the communication is not with the children, but with the parents who make those decisions. And parents have to do that, of course, but on the other hand, often what the kids want or how much they can bear is not considered.

"I saw these kids, so young and yet so afraid of burdening their parents with their own wishes. They didn't want to rock the boat. They saw how much their illness had shattered their families' lives because parents had to spend more time with them and less with their siblings. So they went along with their parents' wishes, because they wanted above all to please their parents.

"We had one little girl, three-and-a-half years old, being treated for a neuroblastoma. She had already had one eye removed, and she was very dehydrated and sick from months of aggressive chemotherapy. Her mom, who was single, had three other kids at home by themselves and had lost her job because she had to stay with her little girl. This child said to me, 'I wish they would stop. I just

The debate over prolonging life at all costs versus dying in peace and dignity continues today, for both children and adults. As the average lifespan increases (a child born by the middle of the twenty-first century can reasonably expect to reach the age of ninety-five), our nation's culture views dying as a disease in search of a cure. We obsessively value quantity over quality of life. The inevitable process of death is used to sell products, push political agendas, and support various religious perspectives. It doesn't matter whether the management of death is primitive or state of the art — the dying are treated like objects. Medical technology and the fears of relatives often override the wishes of terminal patients to let go.

want to play. I don't want to be sick anymore. If I felt better, Mommy wouldn't have to spend all her time here.'"

A GROWING FEAR

Ricky's training as a nurse gave her many ways (besides humor) to deny the frightening prospect of cancer. "I thought maybe I had some kind of localized infection. I knew something was going on, but I didn't seem to have any cut or external infection, so I thought I might have a backed-up mammary gland or something. It was Friday night, and I'm a nurse, so I thought, I don't want to bother anybody, I'll just wait till in the morning.

"But as the evening went on, I kept looking in the mirror and thinking, I wish the other one would grow, maybe I'd have a cleavage. Then I thought, What's going on here?

"About eleven o'clock, I called my doctor. He said, 'I don't think we should wait. Come on in.'

"I met him in the emergency room. He said, 'I don't like the look of this. I don't know what's going on, but you need to come back for an ultrasound and mammogram and an MRI. And we probably need to biopsy this thing.' So I went home, and on Saturday morning I had an ultrasound and then a fine needle aspiration.

"It was Tuesday before I got my diagnosis: most likely a phyllodes tumor about six centimeters in size. Phyllodes tumors may be benign or malignant. These tumors may reach a large size, distort the breast and the overlying skin. In some cases, they lead to necrosis of the skin and cause its ulceration.

"The next question was, was it malignant? Two more days, and the answer came

Most cancers of the breast fall into one of two major categories: ductal or lobular carcinoma. Carcinoma is the medical term for cancer that arises in organ tissue, such as lung, breast, colon, and so on. Ductal carcinoma, of which there are multiple subtypes, develops in the ducts of breast tissue. Lobular carcinoma, which occurs far less frequently, originates in glandular tissue or in a breast lobe.

back: malignant, but it hadn't spread. No regional lymph node in-volvement. I was lucky. I had found it early enough. But none of the oncologists in town — I knew most of them; I had worked with 90 percent of the doctors in my region — had ever seen this kind of tumor in a woman of my age, and they didn't know quite what to do."

HARD CHOICES

"The important thing was to get it out, of course. But should I go through chemotherapy or radiation? Four oncologists gave me four different opinions, everything from a total mastectomy to watchful waiting after a wide excision of the tumor. So I went to the University of Washington and did some research of my own. (This was before the Internet was so accessible; I wish I had had some of the technology that's available today.) I found a single article about a study population of women my age which said that, as long was there was no lymph node involvement, re-section and radiation with fre-quent reexamination was a good risk for women my age. And that's what I chose to do.

"My surgery left me with modest scar tissue and benign fibrocystic changes, with a deep concave distortion on my left side. A year after the opera-tion, I had a saline implant put in to

Like Fern, Ricky had to be assertive and take control of her treatment decision. By exercising medical self-responsibility, she was doing the wise thing. Fortunately, today there are compre-hensive Internet cancer resources available to help match up a person's unique cancer profile with current medi-cal science. This allows individuals to ben-efit from the experience of hundreds of cancer patients. Before such sites became available, sifting through the huge array of medical pa-pers and published studies was an overwhelm-ing task. Even as a health care professional who understood the medical terminology, Ricky found the studies contradictory and confusing. She could not determine with confidence the best course of ac-tion. Says Ricky: "Ultimately, to help you sort out your best treatment choices, you must partner with a physi-cian you believe in."

level the playing field, but later I had it taken out. I didn't like the idea of having a foreign object in me, and it made it difficult to do self-exams to check for recurrence."

FEARS

I ask Ricky what was her greatest fear during her battle with cancer. "I was a single parent with two kids, nine and twelve years old," she replies. "Who was going to take care of them if I wasn't able? My ex-husband had remarried and had new children; his new wife was not ready or willing to take my two, and they would be devastated to have to go live with her, but that would be the most likely outcome. The only other option was to tear my kids away from their school, their friends, and go live with my parents 3,000 miles away.

"I didn't share my worst fears with the kids. They knew Mom was having breast surgery, but they didn't know why. I felt the word 'cancer' would have scared them too much. We had some neighbors whose parents had recently died of cancer. I didn't want my children to be afraid all the time that something would happen to me and that they might be abandoned. They're older now, and we're beyond that. My daughter is actually involved in the Locks of Love — a network of high school kids who grow their hair at least ten inches and then donate it for wigs for chemotherapy patients. Of course, I taught her the correct way to do regular breast self-exams and scheduled her first gynecology appointment when she was eighteen.

"My other worst fear was being alone. I didn't really have to be alone, but I'm not one to reach out to support groups. I can run support groups, but I had such a difficult time reaching out to others

Mastectomy is the surgical removal of the entire breast, sometimes including the lining over the chest muscles and some of the axillary (underarm or armpit) lymph nodes. It is an appropriate treatment option for any patient with breast cancer who, for personal reasons, does not wish to preserve the breast or undergo the postoperative radiation therapy that is recommended with breast-conserving surgery.

at the same time. I did speak with a few women by telephone who were referred to me. Unfortunately, I was turned off by our conversations. The women I spoke to were so dependent, so panicked. They had given in to the disease. I wanted to reach through the phone, shake them, and challenge them to fight, not give up. "I just felt like I'm not going to let this get to me. I have so much more ahead of me. I was determined to deal with my disease but not let it rule me.

"In hindsight, I probably could have found women with whom I could have had a different experience; who I could have helped and who would have kept me from feeling so alone. Or a group, where I could have talked about what I was going through — 'Should I have a reconstruction or not?' I could have discussed treatment options with my friends or my family, but I chose not to. I didn't think they were ready, and neither was I."

WALLS

Like many other cancer patients, Ricky found the emotional complications of dealing with friends and loved ones more painful than the physical ordeal of beating the cancer. "I had a lot of things on my mind through this. I put up walls for protection, for coping, and I worked hard to keep life as normal as possible. I kept quiet about my cancer diagnosis and didn't tell many people.

"Since then, my friends have told me how hurt they were that I didn't involve them, and that I had no right to exclude them, to assume they couldn't handle it. They're right, of course. I was wrong to have denied them the chance to be there for me.

"I already knew that family and friends were important, but with this experience, I made a conscious decision to work more at those relationships than I had in the past. To carve out time to stay more actively involved in their lives despite geographic distances — not just quantity, but quality time. And to let them know how very much they mean to me.

"I found that I couldn't drive myself home from the hospital after surgery and treatment sessions. My parents were ready to come out and help, but I wanted to keep them minimally involved until I knew what I was dealing with. I could name ten friends for whom I would have been there in a heartbeat. Even so, it was so hard for me to ask them for help. It was as if I was admitting defeat, in some way. But when I did reach out to my two dearest friends, Christie and Connie, they came immediately, no questions asked, and stayed with me and took care of me. That was hard for me — to just let go and let them take care of me the way I would have taken care of them.

"Even sexually, I've learned to let that special person in my life give to me, just as it gives me pleasure to give to him. It works both ways. That was a really hard lesson I learned, having observed both my parents as constant givers.

"I resolved to express my emotions more in the moment. I thought of all the people I had wanted to say something to at crucial times but didn't — I would let the moment pass and later wish I hadn't. I wanted to heal my relationships with people I didn't treat the way I would want to be treated, so I went to each of them and tried to make peace with them, to put things right."

MAGICAL PURPOSE

"The thing that really changed my whole life, though, was realizing that it could end in a moment. I knew that before my diagnosis, of course, but like everybody else I just assumed I was going to live to a ripe old age. I still think so, but I've decided to live every day to the fullest because it could be my last. To follow my heart, not my head. To listen to my gut, my intuition, when it comes to major decisions. In other words, to think about what really matters, and to live life with more passion. With magical gusto.

"Magical gusto is something we all have inside us, but we get so caught up in the details of daily life — human doings rather than human beings — that we don't learn to use it. There are miracles offered to us in the world every day, but our receptors are down and we don't see them. I don't know who said, 'When the student is ready, the teacher will appear,' but it's true. While driving home from the hospital with the good news that my tumor was localized with no metastasis, I saw my first double rainbow. This was no accident; it was a magical experience, and I felt overwhelmed with tears. I needed to cry since I was so darn stoic and had not shed a tear up to that moment. I felt the floodgates open and the walls around my heart begin to melt. I recall talking with my children that evening with the one intention to emphasize that whatever they do in life — whether it is art, building something, or even a basic chore — do it 150 percent and do it with passion.

"It's important to find your purpose in life. I know my purpose here on this planet at this time is to help others reach their potential. We all have the ability to touch a life and make a difference, and I find that I have the gift to attract and retain talented people and work with them and through them to reach so many other people — at the food bank, or in school, or helping cancer patients."

Ricky finds that the experience of surviving cancer has increased her empathy with other cancer survivors. Like them, she feels things more deeply and tunes in with greater sensitivity. "It sounds crazy, but I can be at a party and, by looking at someone's eyes across the room, find a person who's been touched by cancer. I just know; I can't tell you how. A reporter came up to me after she heard me speak the other day, and we were talking, and I said, 'You've been touched by — are you a survivor yourself?' She said, 'How did you know?'"

> "It's important to find your purpose in life. I know my purpose here on this planet at this time is to help others reach their potential."

LAUGH WITH THE PUNCHES

Ricky knows that having a sense of humor is an important part of coping with cancer. Even in the initial shock of being diagnosed with breast cancer, she found comedy. "When I was diagnosed, and had this one big boob, I said, 'Instead of taking that one off, can't you enlarge the other one?' I kept looking in the mirror sideways, thinking, So this what I've been missing all these years!

"When I had the implant put in, my natural breast was notice-ably smaller than my reconstructed left breast. I looked lopsided. The implant gave me a very robust breast that sort of saluted the clouds. It actually passed the pencil test, despite my having breast-fed my two children. And my right breast, I thought, looked like an old lady's butt. So the question occurred to me, Do I put an implant in the right side? My breasts are sensitive to me sexually, and I had lost that sexual stimulation in the reconstructed breast, so I decided not to get an implant on the right.

"Then I got deeply involved with someone. We could laugh about the situation. After awhile, when we went to make love, he would automatically go for the right side. It became a standing joke — like he had Michael Jackson's right-hand glove."

As it happened, Ricky's decision to have the original implant was repealed a year later by a twist of fate. "I was in a car accident. My left implant ruptured, and I had to have it taken out. Then the ques-tion was, should I put in a new one? And I decided, I am not my breasts. What you see is what you get.

"And it worked out. I've been lifting weights, and I've actually filled out. I'm not as lopsided as I once was. It's evened up more than I ever could have wished for."

For a woman undergoing a mastectomy, the option of reconstruction is very compelling. When a man is diag-nosed with breast cancer, the treatment is pretty straightforward: modified radi-cal mastectomy with no reconstruction. A man may, of course, elect to have reconstruction, but few do so. While the physical nature of breast cancer is virtually identical for men and women, the psychology and sociology are not. In Western soci-eties, a woman's breasts have an exaggerated importance in terms of self-image, sexual desirability, and fashion. The growing-up experience — first trip with mom for a fitting, the profile in the mirror, the teenage boys trying to get to "second base," the two-piece swimsuit, a dress that shows cleavage, bust-enhancing bras — reinforces the social fact that these are important. They serve as a source of pride, shame, or embarrassment, and they need to be protected, flaunted, enhanced, covered, exposed, leveraged, and bargained for.

ADULT CONCERNS

"I've been afraid that my social life would be affected, that people — let's be honest, men — wouldn't want to get involved with me if they knew I had cancer. You know, 'God, I'm single, who's gonna want me now?' A man I went out with got angry because I didn't tell him on our first date. He thought he might get cancer because he had kissed me. "But I've come to accept it. My cancer is part of my life experience, and like other parts of my past, I reveal it when the time is right. Once I get involved with someone, I usually choose to tell him reasonably early so he has an exit strategy. If this is something he gets frightened about or can't deal with, then we need to either talk about it right away or break it off.

"And I've gotten both kinds of reactions. I've had the reaction where the person says nothing immediately, but not long afterward says, 'I just think this isn't gonna work,' and gives vague reasons that don't make sense. Others have said, 'That doesn't change the way I feel. I just don't want to lose you.' And those are the special people who make sure I go for my follow-up visits and are there to lean on when I get scared.

"So I want people to get to know me as *me* before I tell them about my cancer. And then if they can't deal with it, they're not right for me anyway. But I don't want it to be, 'Oh, I heard you're a cancer survivor. That's awful.' I feel so uncomfortable when people feel sorry for me. I don't want people to feel sorry for me.

"I'm not my cancer — I'm me. And I'm great!"

No matter how worldly or sophisticated or independent we think we are, a life crisis tends to remind us that we are part of a greater whole. This is what Thornton Wilder was saying to us in the following passage from Our Town:

Rebecca

I never told you about that letter Jane Crofut got from her minister when she was sick. He wrote Jane a letter and on the envelope the address was like this: It said: Jane Crofut; The Crofut Farm; Grover's Corner; Sutton County; New Hampshire; United States of America.

George

What's funny about that?

Rebecca

But listen, it's not finished: the United States of America; Continent of North America; Western Hemisphere; the Earth; the Solar System; the Universe; the Mind of God — that's what it said on the envelope.

Whether your name is on the building or you are the one who cleans up after everyone else has gone home, you are part of the same universe of emotions and experiences as the rest of us. We grow, learn, give, receive, love, hate, fear, and rejoice as a community. We need and we are needed.

Perhaps the poet John Donne said it most memorably:

> *. . . any man's death diminishes me*
> *because I am involved in mankind*
> *and therefore never send to know for whom the bell tolls;*
> *it tolls for thee.*

7

The Voice of Resilience

NINETEEN-YEAR-OLD DOUG ULMAN, college sophomore, loved soccer. That's one of the reasons he had chosen to leave his familiar Maryland surroundings and go to school in Providence, Rhode Island. "I grew up playing soccer, and I chose Brown University for their reputation for academic excellence and their great soccer program.

"I majored in American history and education and was looking forward to becoming a teacher. I always enjoyed working with kids when I was in high school, whether it was teaching soccer or mentoring or whatever.

"After my freshman year at Brown, I decided that in order to make an impact on the soccer team I was going to have to train really hard." He began running and working out at home in Maryland while on summer vacation.

Doug especially liked to run. It was good training for soccer, and the exercise usually made him feel good. But on this warm August night, after a three-mile run, he didn't feel well at all. His throat tightened up, and he had trouble breathing. Fearing an asthma attack, Doug's parents persuaded him to go to the emergency room.

"If it was up to me, I probably wouldn't have gone, but my parents urged me to go have it checked out. I got a chest X-ray, and the next day my internist read it and saw a suspicious shadow. He didn't know what it was, but on his recommendation I got a CAT scan the following day. That's when they found the growth in my rib cage.

"Since it hadn't caused me any pain, and I wasn't feeling ill, they said, 'No problem, chances are 98 percent it's benign. We'll just take it out and that'll be the end of it.'

"So in the span of a week, I went from running and having a little problem breathing to the emergency room to the CAT scan center to the hospital in Baltimore to have this chest resection. And I came out of surgery fine and returned to fairly normal activity."

But this sudden crisis — as suddenly resolved, it seemed — was only a warmup for what was to come. "About two weeks later I went back with my parents for a checkup before returning to college for my sophomore year. We assumed the doctor was going to check the incision site for infection or scarring. But as soon as we entered his office, he said, 'It's been confirmed. You have cancer. It's cancer of the cartilage, and it's called chondrosarcoma.'"

SUCKER PUNCH

Today Doug can talk calmly about his disease, but that day in the doctor's office, hearing the diagnosis for the first time, Doug stared back at the doctor as through a thick fog. "I was in shock. The possibility of a malignant tumor had not even remotely crossed my mind. My parents were crying in disbelief.

Fifty years ago, a cancer diagnosis was considered an automatic death sentence; science understood little about the disease or how to control it. Today, however, over 60 percent of Americans diagnosed with cancer will live longer than five years, and their chances of long-term survival improve dramatically after the five-year mark. The National Cancer Institute estimates that there are over 8 million Americans who are living with cancer or have been cured. This is due in large part to early detection and quick intervention. The sooner a cancer is found and treated, the better a patient's chance for survival.

However, it's also true that although people of all ages can develop one or more of the over 100 types of cancer, most types are more common in people over the age of fifty. Usually cancer develops gradually over many years, due, it is thought, to a complex mix of nutritional, hereditary, lifestyle, and environmental factors. Doug's cancer, chondrosarcoma, for example, occurs most often in middle-aged and older people, most frequently in the hips and legs. While the causes of cancer are not completely understood, we do know that healthy lifestyle choices can dramatically reduce the risk of developing most cancers. These include not smoking, maintaining a healthy diet, moderate to zero alcohol intake, and moderate exercise.

The doctor talked about the radical surgery he wanted to perform, which was to take out part of my spine and part of my ribs and immobilize my vertebrae. It might mean I wouldn't be able to run or even walk. We weren't just talking about a minor cancer diagnosis. We were looking at a life-changing procedure.

"In one second, everything changed from Geez, I'm going back to school, everything's great, to What do I do now? How does this affect my life? So many thoughts and frustrations and fears and worries. Too many for a nineteen-year-old."

From the distance of a few years, Doug sees the bright side of that dark day. "Lucky for me, because I had spent the summer working out and exercising, I was probably in the best shape I've ever been in, both mentally and physically, when I was diagnosed. I ran five miles the day before my surgery. I wasn't sick or in pain, and that's partly why the doctors thought the tumor would be benign.

"In fact, if I hadn't been exercising, it's conceivable that we wouldn't have found out about the cancer, because my breathing problem was unrelated. That tumor would still be growing inside me today if I hadn't gone to the emergency room that night, and it might not have caused me any pain until twenty years from now, because it's such a slow-growing tumor. Doctors aren't positive, but they say it could have been there for six or seven years."

DEALING WITH THE REALITY

Doug and his parents wisely decided to consult other doctors and see if a less radical, less disabling treatment was possible. "It was a slow-growing tumor, so we didn't feel the urgency to jump right in. So we came home and regrouped.

"One of my first thoughts was, Oh, I'm not going back to school. I remember telling my dad, and he came into my room later and said, 'You know, you're welcome to stay home, and it's fine if you want to take this semester off, but all your friends are going to be at school, and no one's going to be here, and you'll end up just sitting around.' I decided to go back to school, and that was probably the best decision I ever made — to be around my friends, my support system.

"The next day, we packed the car. I was still on painkillers from the surgery and couldn't drive, so my mom drove me from Baltimore to Providence. I tried to live as normal a life as possible under the circumstances, but it was difficult. For the next several weeks it was a long, slow process of sending films and charts to different doctors and trying to get second opinions.

"It can be frustrating to be nineteen years old and trying to communicate with doctors, and the doctors are communicating with your parents. Especially since I was in Rhode Island and they were in Baltimore. A lot of what I heard was secondhand.

"The doctor who gave me the cancer diagnosis was a surgeon, and he seemed to think I needed surgery right away. But the oncologists we consulted didn't think it was that urgent. In fact, the one we were most comfortable with recommended that we do nothing. This was a relief, but it was confusing. It seemed we had two options: do nothing, or have radical surgery with major side effects.

"A doctor in New York broke the tie. He agreed that waiting was the way to go. We finally settled on an oncologist in Baltimore who explained the situation to us. He told us, 'The chance of recurrence is less than 50 percent, so let's wait and watch it. If the chances were above 50 percent, we might do the surgery as a precaution. But since it's slow-growing, we can watch it and if it comes back then at least we all know that surgery is the next step.' We were comfortable with that. He's still my oncologist today, and it's been three years since the original diagnosis, and nothing has shown up so far, so I'm pretty happy with our decision."

NEW CONCERNS

Unfortunately, the chondrosarcoma was not the only health problem Doug would have to contend with. The following February, at home for a long weekend, Doug went to see his internist. "He examined me and did some blood work, and he noticed a mole on my chest. He said, 'You know, you might want to have that checked out.' I have a fair number of moles, and this one didn't look unusual to me, but it had a red spot in it that the internist noticed.

"I went to my dermatologist, who removed the mole. She also referred me to a national dermatology clinic at Johns Hopkins where, she said, 'a lot of different doctors and a lot of different eyes can view you.'

"After my visit to Johns Hopkins, I went back to school and started studying and playing soccer and totally forgot about the mole. One night I was in my room getting ready to go to soccer practice when the dermatologist called. She said, 'Remember that mole we took off two weeks ago?' I said, 'Yeah.' She said, 'Well, it's malignant melanoma.'"

The numb feeling, the shock Doug had experienced in the doctor's office was back. "She told me more about it, but to be honest, I don't remember much of that conversation. I remember her saying the words 'malignant melanoma' and telling me I needed to have more surgery because they were worried that it could have spread.

"I ended up going to soccer practice that night. The dermatologist had already called my mom, and my mom had called my coach and told him about it in case I showed up acting strange or in a bad mood. I remember telling some of the guys on the team, 'Hey, I'm having more surgery.' They asked questions, and I couldn't answer most of them because I didn't know much about melanoma.

"I flew home the next week to have the area re-excised. And the more I learned about it, the scarier it got. I had gotten comfortable with what we had decided to do with the chondrosarcoma, just waiting and watching and getting CAT scans, and now I was being told about a disease called melanoma, for which

Facts about melanoma:

- At current rates, one in 74 Americans will develop melanoma during his or her lifetime.
- There will be about 47,700 new cases of melanoma in 2000.
- In 2000, 7,700 deaths will be attributed to melanoma — 4,800 men and 2,900 women — a death rate of nearly one per hour.
- Older Caucasian males have the highest mortality rates from melanoma.
- The incidence of melanoma more than tripled among Caucasians between 1980 and 2000.

Source: American Cancer Society

there were no blood tests and no markers and no way to tell what was actually going on. That's why so many people die from melanoma — often the first sign is getting ill from lymph node metastasis. I've since learned that 50 percent of melanomas are found by patients and 50 percent by doctors. That's why skin self-exams are so important.

"So it was starting all over again. I thought I knew all I needed to know about cancer, but I didn't know anything about melanoma, and although chondrosarcoma and melanoma are both called cancer, they're really two very different diseases."

Back again were the fear and anger he had experienced after his first diagnosis. "The anger was in asking myself, Why me? And wondering, What did I do wrong? How did I get this? It takes a while to get past that, and once you do, your recovery speeds up exponentially. You realize, hey, it's not just me, it's 1.2 million people, and they're young and old and black and white and male and female, and there's no discrimination.

"The fear, the first time, was of the unknown — What's going to happen to me? What does this mean for the future? But the second time, it was, Is it going to come back? Has it spread? This was a lot scarier than the first time because of the nature of melanoma itself.

"After the re-excision, I got some good news: the melanoma was encapsulated, which meant it didn't have the characteristics needed to spread. The bad news was that once you have melanoma, the chances of having a recurrence go up. I asked the doctor, 'How are we going to know?' She looked at me and said, 'Well, we just wait and see and watch and take pictures of the skin and look for changes.'

"This isn't very comforting when you're dealing with the

Melanoma leaves its host ever vigilant. Regardless of how one spot turns out, the next one may well be bad news. Any good news you get is tempered by the knowledge that diligent self-exams and professional screenings will always be a part of your life. The irony is that you hope this just-below-the-surface fear and routine screening annoyance lasts for many, many years.

deadliest form of cancer. I said to myself, I'm not going to die in the next five years, or in the next ten years, but at some point this disease is going to catch up with me — if not melanoma, then another kind of cancer — and I won't be so lucky in catching it early next time. That feeling lasted awhile, but later I realized that if I kept a positive attitude I could beat it."

A WARNING ITCH

About three months later, doctors found another melanoma on Doug's skin. "Most of the literature on melanomas shows these grotesque-looking things, and people look at the pictures and say, 'Oh, if it doesn't look like that, then it can't be melanoma.' But that's not the case.

"I returned home from school in the middle of May and went to my dermatologist for a checkup. She looked at several moles and said, 'Nothing looks that bad. Are any of them bothering you?' I showed her one on my upper left arm that was small and flat and light brown; it didn't look unusual, but it itched. She said, 'Well, it looks fine. It's flat, and it's symmetrical. But if it's been itching, let's take it off.' She just scraped off the top layer of skin and put in a few stitches.

"Ten days later I went in to get the stitches removed. Usually the nurse does this, and you don't even see the doctor. But the nurse said, 'The doctor wants to see you.' I waited two hours, and I began to worry. Finally they took me to an examination room, and the door opened, and four doctors came in. And I knew we didn't need four doctors to take out the stitches.

"My doctor said that the mole had come back as invasive melanoma, which right off the bat didn't sound too good. And she had brought in these other doctors to explain the different treatment options. The first step was to re-excise, because she had only scraped off the top of the tumor, and they needed to find out how deep it had gone and whether it had spread. They said, 'Look, the first one you had was bad, but we were able to take it out, and that one will never come back. But this one is a bit more worrisome, because not only has it had the opportunity to spread, but it could recur anywhere.'

"I was overwhelmed. There I was, by myself, facing four doctors who were giving me all this information that I couldn't write down or even think about. I was shocked and upset and frustrated. But I wasn't totally surprised, because I had half expected to get it again.

"My parents were returning that night from an Alaska cruise, and I went to pick them up at the airport. They were telling me how great their trip was, and I didn't know how to tell them my news because I didn't want to ruin their good feelings. But I told them, and the first thing my mom did when she got home was call the doctor. That was good, because then I got to listen with a clear head.

"So I had a re-excision for this mole. They went very deep to be sure they got it all, and there was no sign of spreading to the nearby lymph nodes. Again I felt fortunate. I was lucky it had itched.

"The day scheduled for the surgery for this mole was, ironically, the day after our first Ulman Cancer Fund fundraiser. I remember telling people that the next day I was undergoing surgery for the scariest cancer I've had."

Any parent with a child at risk will tell you that, even when you're continents apart, your child is always with you. As a parent, you finance medical care and oversee medical decisions, of course, but there's something else you provide that is crucial: a normal life, or as close to normal as possible. With a grown-up child on the brink of independence, you must do this without smothering or overprotecting. You need to move on with your life today and encourage your child to do the same, and not be stopped by the unknowable tomorrow. Cancer is a reminder: your business in life is to live, not to die; to stay in school, to keep playing soccer, to go on vacation — to appreciate what you can do, and do it.

CHANCES OF A LIFETIME

At the age of twenty-three, Doug feels he's been blessed with opportunities most people will never have: the opportunity to beat cancer several times, the opportunity to establish a foundation to help other people, the opportunity to speak to children and young adults about cancer prevention and detection.

One special opportunity stands out in Doug's mind — a chance to run a marathon in the Himalayas. "Other people were thinking how hard it [the marathon] was; I spent a lot of my time there thinking how fortunate I was to be able to do it. And I thought about all the other cancer survivors I've come in contact with who may or may not be able to accomplish such a physical feat. I said to myself, You know, part of this is doing it for them and doing it with the knowledge that you're lucky to be able to return to a normal life — although other people say it's an abnormal life, because it's above and beyond a normal life. It was such a personal accomplishment, physically and emotionally, to be able to say, Hey, I've been slowed down three times now, and three years later, I'm back!

"I'm going to live a full, normal life. I have no doubt of that, although I did waver a little between diagnoses. There's no doubt in my mind that I'll live to eighty or ninety. And I'll live a much more fulfilled life than most people my age. Life is better the second time. I wouldn't trade my experience for anything in the world. It's made me think in a way that many twenty-two-year-olds don't think, and it's something that's reinforced every day when I watch other people my age go through cancer.

"My friend lost his mom last week to cancer, and I watched him go through the same emotions. I asked myself, Isn't there some way that we can change this so that people don't have to go through the exact same thing? But there's no way to do that. Until you experience something like this yourself, it's hard to know what it's like. And it's a shame that something negative has to happen in order for people to find out how special each day and each second is.

Between discoveries, Doug sought the support of other young cancer survivors but found that, although there were support groups for specific types of cancer and groups that focused on small children, there was really nothing for young adults. Doug had discovered his mission and purpose. In 1997, he founded the Ulman Cancer Fund for Young Adults (www.ulmanfund.org), whose mission is to provide support programs, education, and resources, free of charge, to benefit young adults and their families and friends who are affected by cancer, and to promote awareness and prevention of cancer.

"It's taught me that no one is immune from disease or illness, from things that are intrusive and scary. And it's taught me that you don't have to let these things control your life. It's reinforced the importance of family, and of truly taking advantage of life. It's reminded me that so many things in life are unimportant, and that so many of the ways you can spend your life are meaningless. I can't imagine ever going back to the way I was, not realizing these things."

GOING FOR THE GOAL

"I'm going to ride my bike twenty miles this afternoon, which will be the longest ride I've ever done. Next weekend, I'm going to Texas to ride a hundred-mile race, a fundraiser for cancer. A friend who's going with me said, 'Geez, it's going to be so hard.' I said, 'Do you have any doubt you're going to finish it?' She said, 'No.' I said, 'Then it doesn't matter how hard it is, if you don't think about it. Think about all the people who wished they could be doing it, and all the people who are going to benefit from it. You'll have no problem finishing it. And when you do, you'll realize that it's just something you never dreamed you could do.'

"I've come to realize that I can't perform in any capacity without having goals. As soon as I finished the marathon in Las Vegas, I had to set a goal to do this bike ride. It gives me something to work for, and when I accomplish it, it's that much more special because I've been focusing on it for so long. One goal I set was getting healthy again. After my first chest surgery, the doctor told me it would be six weeks before I could start training to play soccer again. I set that as a goal. I put on my soccer uniform and sat on the field. I visualized myself running, practicing, playing soccer. I checked off every single day on my calendar, and at the end of six weeks I started running. Two weeks later I started practicing for soccer, and two weeks after that I played in a game.

"If we don't set goals that seem unachievable, then we'll never live life the way it's intended to be lived."

"If we don't set goals that seem unachievable, then we'll never live life the way it's intended to be lived."

"THE GOOD KIND"

"About a year after I was diagnosed, I was coaching some seven-year-olds at a soccer camp. During a lunch break, one of the kids asked me, 'How are you doing?' And I said, 'Fine.' He said, 'Is your cancer all gone?' I said, 'Yes.' And he said, 'Oh, well, you must have had the good kind.' I said, 'What do you mean?' And he said, 'Well, my grandfather had the bad kind and that's the kind when you can't live anymore afterwards.' And I thought, Geez, that's the way his parents explained it to him. It took me a while to think whether that was good or bad, but in the end I decided, hey, that's not a bad way to think about it."

Twenty-three, just embarking on his adult life, and diagnosed with cancer — not once, but three times. A young athlete, full of promise, cut down in the prime of his powers. A sad story, yes?

Then why is Doug not crying?

It's quite obvious, when you hear him tell his story, just how positive and optimistic Doug is. He gives thanks for the lessons his cancers have taught him — lessons about setting implausible goals, living affirmatively, challenging difficulty head-on. Although he expects to live a normal life span, he refuses to confine himself to a normal life. He recognizes that negative emotions are a temporary but normal reaction to bad news, and that a positive attitude over the long run, in pursuit of long-range goals, is what counts.

Not only does Doug's attitude make him an inspiration to those around him, it keeps him healthier than he might otherwise be. The wisest among us have known for centuries that body and mind are two aspects of the same being and thus inseparable. Medical research confirms this wisdom. Recent scientific studies have shown that our thoughts, our feelings, our attitudes toward life and its difficulties strengthen the immune system and profoundly affect the healing power of the body. When the body and mind are in full communication, the body can achieve the goals set by the mind.

We think of medicine as science and living as art. There is no more reason for this dichotomy than the mythical divide between body and mind. Medical science encompasses the art of the doctor's bedside manner, the patient's positive outlook, the family's and community's role in nursing a patient back to health. The art of living well includes paying attention to the science of lowering health risk factors, keeping up with advances in medicine, and giving yourself positive recovery instructions.

Like his hero Lance Armstrong, Doug Ulman demonstrates the art and science of living life in full.

8

The Voice of the Spirit

IN 1991, PAULA KOSKEY WAS GETTING USED TO BEING A SINGLE MOM, a widow of four years, working to support three children — two sons, fourteen-year-old Jesse and eight-year-old Luke, and a daughter, HopeAnne, twelve. "When my husband and I had our kids, we made the decision that I would be a full-time homemaker. So I was going through the adjustment of getting back into the work force. I was working as a secretary. I was running two or three miles every day. Life was good. I was beginning to get the balance back in my life, and it was a very fine time. Occasionally, I felt tired — but what forty-year-old single mother doesn't feel tired?

"One night, lying in bed, I discovered I had this lump at the base of my neck — a little, grape-sized lump. It wasn't painful. I didn't think anything of it. It was a surprise, but not a major concern.

"I was working at Providence Hospital, and I had decided to switch departments. I was accepted for a new position, but the director I was working for decided to keep me for the full thirty days, as the rules allowed, before releasing me to the new department.

"I figured that I would get all the medical tests I needed before going to the new job. One of the things I needed was a visit with a gynecologist. While I was in her office, sitting on the edge of the table — this is crystal clear in my memory — I debated with myself whether to say something about the lump, even though it wasn't her specialty.

"I decided to ask her about it. She didn't do a needle biopsy — she just felt it. And I immediately got an inkling that something was wrong when she asked, 'Who is your surgeon?'

"It got scarier. By the time my appointment was over, she had already made arrangements for me to see a surgeon that day. That kind of freaked me out.

"So I visited the surgeon. He set up an appointment to do a biopsy. And here's my one claim to fame: on the very day I started my new job — in the cancer center — I learned I had cancer. Hodgkin's lymphoma."

The shock of that day will always be in her memory. Now, nine years later, she can joke about it:

"Every day since that day, I get down on my knees and thank God I didn't start working for the morgue!"

GIVING AND RECEIVING SUPPORT

Cancer has a way of taking control of your daily life and resetting your priorities. Paula and her doctors immediately started testing and deciding and scheduling, and Paula began to deal with the implications of her disease for her family. "The oncologist said it was probably stage one or two, nothing to be really concerned about. I'd probably have some more tests and then radiation. So I started going through the paces for the tests, and by the time I was done, they had determined that I was stage three. That means that the cancer involves lymph node groups above and below the diaphragm. I would have to go through chemotherapy."

Hodgkin's disease is a rare cancer that develops in the lymphatic system, a part of the body's circulatory system that helps fight disease and infection. It accounts for only 1 percent of all cancer cases in the United States. The most common symptom is a painless swelling in the lymph nodes under the arm or in the neck or groin.

Any single parent — especially the parent of children whose other parent has died — knows the deep, primitive fear children have that they will be left alone in the world. Paula knew she would have to reassure her kids, but that hiding the truth, the possibility that they might lose her too, would only heighten their apprehension. Paula had a certain degree of control over her life, as well as the rigor and routine of treatment to fill her days. Her children had a much more difficult task: they could only watch helplessly and hope for the best.

"Like a lot of people, I could cope well during the day, because I had to. I had three young kids, and I wasn't going to let it affect them any more than it had to. But I would wake up in the middle of the night, and that's when I'd cry. So I started keeping a journal, and that's when I'd let the thoughts come out. Thoughts like, 'I could die.' Of course, I knew I could die — we all do.

"I didn't want to make any promises to my children that this was going to be fine, because I didn't know. What I did tell them is that I was going to do everything possible to beat the disease. And that's all I could promise them. I didn't put it in those words exactly, but I was very open with them, just as I've been their whole lives.

"My kids were a blessing. Jeff, my oldest son, handled it very well. He would listen to me a lot. I tried to be careful, because I didn't want to burden him, but he would listen, and that was wonderful. I think he's always been mature for his age anyway. Luke, my youngest, would bring me aspirin. Initially, HopeAnne, my middle child, had a hard time and was really suffering. Some days, going through chemo was nothing compared with handling her reaction. She had already lost one parent, and she knew that if I died, that would be it. And her reaction was to completely withdraw from it, and from me. If I went to touch her, she would pull away from me. It was tough for me, very painful. We are very close now, but that was a scary time for her and it was tough and painful for me.

"Outside the home, everyone was so supportive. I received nearly a hundred cards during my

Paula's doctors at first thought they had detected her Hodgkin's disease early, in stage one or stage two. "Staging" is simply a way to describe the extent of a cancer, using such characteristics as the size of the tumor, lymph node involvement, and where it has spread. Systems of staging have been custom-designed for specific cancers. Usually staging is by number — the larger the number, the more advanced the disease. However, it may simply be termed "localized" (confined to the primary site), "metastatic" (spread to other areas of the body), or "recurrent" (cancer that has returned in its original site or occurred in another part of the body after treatment).

treatment, and I tacked them all to my wall. It was wonderful to go to bed and see them — like looking at a wall full of hugs.

"My Dad would come over after my chemo to see if I needed anything. My sister-in-law and her husband would take my kids on weekends. People at work would make meals for me. My father-in-law, who was doing a stint with the Peace Corps, took a leave and came to our house to care for the kids and me during my last month of chemo.

"My very best friend and I rode to work together, and when I was having chemo she would give me a ride home. She could keep everything in perspective for me. I would have chemo on Thursday and work the rest of the day because I wouldn't feel the effects until Friday. Friday was a tough day, but she would make me laugh, because she'd say things like, 'Uh-oh, you're green, it's time to go.'

"I felt richer than I had felt in a long, long time. Not that I ever felt unloved, but this was far more intense than I had ever felt before. I was never unaware of my blessings. Before my cancer diagnosis, I was thankful for the day, for the little things. When I would run, I would be thankful that I was able to run. I was already smelling the roses before this happened. Just not as intensely."

HAIR

People undergoing cancer treatment often experience alopecia — the falling out of some or all of the head hair, sometimes in clumps on the pillow in the morning, usually during shampooing or brushing. In most cases it grows back, but in the meantime, heaped on top of the pain and nausea of treatment, it's a demoralizing blow to the spirit, an insult to one's self-esteem, and many patients try to hide the damage.

"People told me, 'You need to get a wig, because you're going to be doing drugs that will make all your hair fall out.' They told me I should do it while I still had my hair, so I could match my color and style.

"I went wig shopping, but I couldn't go through with it. I would try on a wig and then just start sobbing. I knew that wasn't the right way for me to handle it. I decided instead I was going to wear a hat, and if people couldn't deal with my naked head, that was their problem. "My sister-in-law came over one night with a bottle of wine and gave me a buzz cut. So my youngest son and I had matching hair, and that was okay with me. Later, when my hair started falling out, it wasn't as devastating as if it had been long strands of hair.

Give me a head with hair;
long, beautiful hair. Shining, gleaming, flaxen, waxing. . . .
there's just no words for the beauty, the splendor, and the wonder of my hair.

From the song "Hair"

It's normal for men and women to feel distressed about hair loss. Hair helps to distinguish us in a crowded world. It lets us express opinions and emotions — short hair, long hair, purple hair, green hair, mohawks, shaved-in initials, braids, beads, ponytails, and, of course, the more-noticeable-than-they-realize comb-overs.

Military recruits are routinely buzzed clean the first day of basic training. This is done, in part, to minimize the spread of head lice, but it's also a way of neutralizing individual personalities. The young soldier goes in looking like cocky and confident Sam Muntzel from Buffalo and comes out feeling naked and looking like one of a thousand GI Joes. This initial feeling of vulnerability and embarrassment is the same for most cancer patients who lose their hair. It helps to understand why it happens, and to know that hair will grow back.

The healthy scalp contains approximately 100,000 hairs, constantly growing, with old hairs falling out and being replaced by new ones. Hair loss occurs because chemotherapy drugs travel throughout the body to kill cancer cells, and some of these drugs damage hair follicles, causing the hair to fall out. Not all patients experience this, and not all chemotherapy drugs cause it. Some drugs can cause hair loss over the entire body; others affect only the scalp. Radiation therapy to the head often causes scalp hair loss, and sometimes, depending on the dose, the hair thus lost does not regrow naturally.

If hair loss does occur, it usually begins within two weeks of the start of therapy, and gets worse one to two months after the start of therapy. Hair regrowth often begins even before therapy is completed.

"One day at work I looked down at some papers on my desk, touched my head, and watched my hair fall on the pages like little snowflakes.

"I got very angry. I kicked the filing cabinet. I left the building and ran around in the parking lot. But God is very smart, because I never lost all my hair. I think He knew He didn't want to put up with me if I had to go through that kind of ordeal. It wasn't that I was really angry with God, I was just angry because I didn't want to be in this situation. And as the treatments went on, the anger dissipated. It didn't last. And I never did the 'Why me?' thing.

"As for the hair, I turned into one of those guys whose hair is all lined up, you know? I'd get up in the morning and literally arrange my hair. I maintained this façade of having a somewhat full head of hair. And that was okay. I worked in the cancer center, and it was a very accepting atmosphere.

"I wore a hat to work every day. I was sitting in my office one evening, and the work day was over, and my oncologist, Dr. Terebelo, walked in. We would occasionally chat, not about what I was going through, just things in general. And he said, 'What's up with the hat?' I told him, this is what I'm going to do. And he just looked at me and said, 'You know, you don't have to do that.' That was probably one of the nicest things anybody had ever said to me."

THE GOOD DOCTOR

Paula was grateful for the kindness, competence, and compassion of her oncologist. In this book you've met a few doctors you wouldn't want you or your family to be subjected to. These are the exceptions; most doctors do their best work with their heart, like Dr. Terebelo.

"Dr. Terebelo and I had a very interesting relationship; we worked together in the cancer center, but I was also his patient. I thought that he probably was equally kind and sensitive with all of his patients, but I certainly felt that he really cared about me as a person. I wasn't the forty-year-old with Hodgkin's, I was Paula."

The conservative chemotherapy Paula started out on proved inadequate, and Dr. Terebelo recommended using more aggressive chemicals. Paula knew this could cause more severe long-term side effects, and she resisted. "When the doctor told me I wasn't responding to my chemo, it hit me that

May 28th, 1992

Dear Dr. Terebelo,

I'm tempted to say I want to thank you now that it's over, but I know it's not. I know that for the next year, while most of me is laughing and enjoying, a part of me will hold back and watch from the shadows and pray. But enough!

I chose you as my physician because I heard you were good and that's what I was looking for. I wanted someone who really knew his stuff, would give me the facts, be a clinician and leave me alone. I was tough. I could handle anything. Thank you for knowing your stuff, being a clinician — and not leaving me alone.

Thank you for trying to educate me. When I was told I had cancer, I felt as though I had suddenly lost control over my own life. (Perhaps because I had?) The only way I could even begin to cope was to learn. Thank you for letting me have access to everything, for being honest and for teaching me — or at least trying!

Thank you for saying I wasn't a wimp, for helping me realize that there is a difference between resting and quitting.

I'd like to say thanks for the medicine, but I'm not quite that masochistic. What I will say is thanks for all the time you spent helping me deal with the medicine. I was always amazed that every time I was in your office, you never seemed rushed. Even when I behaved like a brat, you sat patiently and listened. Thank you for giving so freely of your time.

Thank you for understanding the tears. I tried to tell myself it was okay to cry, but I hated the tears. I was just so scared. Never have I felt so frightened, frustrated or helpless. Thanks for letting me cry and still hold onto my dignity. (I still regret not having stock in Kleenex.)

Thanks for all the pats and handshakes — touch can be healing, too.

Thanks for trying to teach me patience. (I think it may be a lost cause.)

And, no matter what the future holds, thanks so much for doing your best, for knowing that, especially when I'm scared, I need to be involved.

Thanks for arguing with me when it really mattered. (Those closest to me think you are quite brave.)

Love, Paula

I could really die. Up to that time I had not allowed the thought to enter my consciousness. I said, 'It's only been three months, let's just stick with this.'

"He spent two hours talking to me, handing me Kleenexes, saying, 'You know I can't let you make that decision. You have to trust me on this.' Finally he wore me down. He said, 'I'll make a deal with you. Just do it once.' And that's the approach we took, and of course we did it more than once, but he was willing to listen to me and he knew me well enough to know just what to say. He couldn't just say, 'I'm the doctor, and you're gonna do this,' and I couldn't just blindly say, 'Well, okay.' He respected the fact that I needed to be involved.

"I thought, I need to have a game plan. So I got an attorney to make out my will. I had to take care of guardianship for my kids, and I wanted to make sure my affairs were in order. I wrote a farewell poem to my friends.

"Then I made a great turnaround. It was like, Yeah, okay, I could die, but I'm livin'. And from that point on, everything just got better, even though I felt worse, even though the chemo regimen got more and more difficult.

"I didn't actually forecast anything. I simply put myself in God's hands, and I said, 'You know what, do with me what you will, but give me the strength to handle it.' And that's what I did. I just prayed for strength and grace. I think God knew better than to remove me right at that point."

GIVING BACK

It's no surprise that Paula has found satisfaction in helping others get through the ordeal she has survived.

"I'm involved with the Healing Art Center at the hospital. As I said before, when I was first being treated, I was showered with blessings, and I felt a huge need to pay that back. Then, as time went on, I felt a need for someone else to take over. I didn't want to be Paula the cancer survivor, I wanted to be Paula, the person. So I've tried to pull away, but I can't, because I still feel connected, I still feel a need to give back.

"Something has kept me involved. There's so much going on. I wrote a little children's book when my kids were younger, and when I was going through treatment I told my boss I'd like to take my book and give all the proceeds to the cancer center. She said fine. The book, *Secrets of Christmas,* was published by the hospital and raised over $10,000. Then I got something published in *Coping* magazine, and after that I heard from *Chicken Soup* and got involved in some local cancer events."

I asked Paula what discoveries she made and what lessons she learned from this experience.

"What lessons did I learn? Probably the hardest thing I had to learn was acceptance. Not necessarily acceptance of the disease, but acceptance of what people had to offer me, what they wanted to give me. I've always been a doer, I've always been the one giving, and it was very hard for me to learn how to accept gracefully — to come to terms with losing control over things.

"I realized how ironic cancer treatment is. If I go to a bad restaurant and get sick and feel like a Mack truck hit me, and realize it's because of what I ate, chances are I'm not gonna go back there again. I could say, 'Okay, maybe it was something else,' and go back and try it again, but if it happened two times in a row I'd never go back. But I was going in for chemo, and it was like the worst kind of food poisoning, the worst kind of flu, and doggone if I didn't go back two weeks later and do it again. It would knock me off my feet, and just when I was beginning to feel well again, I'd go right back. What kind of silliness is that? It's the direct opposite of everything my mother taught me.

"I was forty, and I got to learn a lot of the stuff you might learn when you're seventy, eighty, ninety."

"I also came to believe drugs were good. Before all this, I avoided taking even an aspirin. By the end of my chemo, I was happy to take my Ativan. Just kind of . . . 'Bring on the drugs!'

"If there's anything I have to be thankful for, it's the intensity of a beautiful and revealing time in my life. I was forty, and I got to learn a lot of the stuff you might learn when you're seventy, eighty, ninety. It gave me a better perspective on life than I normally would have had.

"I was fortunate to have good listeners. There's a very dear friend of mine who was diagnosed with breast cancer five years before I was diagnosed with Hodgkin's. She was like an old pro, and we could talk and laugh with each other about it. And she would listen. People need to remember just to listen. Sometimes silence is one of the greatest gifts there is. You don't have to fill space with sound.

"I also learned about relative pain and discomfort. A year and a half after I was done with chemo for Hodgkin's, I had some abnormal cells in a Pap smear, and my gynecologist said, 'You need a hysterectomy. We're not going to play any games.' I had the hysterectomy, and it was nothing. I did nine long months of chemo, feeling terrible most of the time, a little worse every day. When I had my hysterectomy, I started feeling better the next day.

"One other thing: food. With the first regimen of chemotherapy, I learned to subsist on yogurt and bananas and chocolate and Diet Pepsi. But with the more aggressive chemo, I couldn't eat tomatoes, couldn't eat cheese, couldn't have cola, no bananas, no yogurt, no chocolate. And I'm a chocoholic. So I'd be counting down the days in a two-week cycle till I could have that chocolate bar, and I would enjoy every single bite of it.

"I lost a lot of weight. I never realized it before, but there is such a thing as too thin. That's kind of a cool thing. Now I want to try too rich!"

*Paula is already rich, and
she knows it. In the November/December 1994 issue of*
Coping, *a magazine for cancer survivors, she wrote God the following note:*

*Hey, God (this is the way God and I talk to each other), please bless all my
family and friends, and have a seat, because there's a whole list of stuff for
which I'm grateful.*

*Thank you, God, for my kids. They're such neat people! They have big feet,
but I guess that's so they will make it on this rough road. They sure do seem*

to be walking in the right direction. And they keep bringing me stuff. They bring me aspirin and pop and hugs . . . and smiles to my soul.

Thank you, God, for my family and friends. They change roles so often! Sometimes the people in my family are my closest friends, and sometimes my friends are my closest family. Even though we're related, I must admit these people are very funny looking. They have extraordinarily big ears and shoulders, and hearts! Is that so I don't wear them out when I need someone to listen or cry on or care?

Thank you, God, for my neighbors and co-workers. I'm amazed at how many really wonderful people there are in the world. Sometimes I feel better just seeing their smiles, and all the kind things they do with their hands actually touch my heart.

So thank you, God, for all this good stuff, and bless us. Somehow, I seem to be seeing things in a whole new way. I know there will be more tears, but I also know that tears come from both crying and laughing. Some things can take my hair, drain my body, strain my mind, but nothing can touch my spirit! Thank you for the challenges you've sent my way, and thank you for the people to share the tears. It's nice to see the love.

P.S. Dear God — A few things I forgot:

Thank you for my hair, for however long it lasts. And thanks for letting it grow back.

Thanks for sunglasses. My friends will need them to guard against the chrome-dome glare.

Thank you for computers. They make both work and group letters a whole lot easier.

Thanks for James Taylor. I like the way he sings to me.

Thank you for plants and flowers. They're a nice reminder of spring.

Thanks for men, though I'm not exactly sure why. . . .

Thanks for Diet Pepsi, one thing I can enjoy without the fear of getting fat.

Thanks for chocolate. It's more thrilling than Diet Pepsi and safer than men.

Amen.

9

The Voice of Leadership

I WALK INTO HANK PORTERFIELD'S OFFICE IN HINSDALE, ILLINOIS. He is on the phone, but he smiles and gestures for me to take a seat. I look around the spacious office and see decades of awards and certificates. He is a successful entrepreneur, a businessman of forty years with an engineering degree, an accomplished organizer and leader of men. Now he is the chairman of US TOO! International, the world's largest prostate cancer support group. Hank is a doer, not just a talker.

He finishes the call, stands up — he is tall and thin, in his early seventies — smiles a salesman's smile, and extends his left hand for me to shake. For the next two hours we talk about Hank, his "guys," the importance of attitude, and the role of support groups.

Hank's first encounter with serious illness happened when he was working in Boston as a district sales manager with a mechanical engineering degree. Hank was stricken with polio. He was not yet thirty, and he was the father of four young sons.

"My family was very understanding. I was pretty damn concerned that they were going to come down with it, but they didn't. I fought my way through that and ended up with only a residual weakness in my right shoulder and arm. Two years later I had a medical procedure that alleviated the problem. Aside from the fact that I can't play some of the sports I used to play, it hasn't affected me a whole lot. I liked to play ball with the boys, and I had to learn to throw as a lefty.

"When I was called back to the home office in the Midwest, the boys weren't very happy about having to leave their friends. So I promised them we would buy a farm, and that's what we did. I continued in the advertising end of my company's business and became manager of distributor sales. But after we had been there five or six years, another company hired me and we had to move back to Massachusetts. And some time after that, I had another job offer that brought me to Chicago.

"I worked for that company for a while, then I went into the real estate business in the western suburbs. In the '80s I ended up in commercial real estate, buying apartment complexes until the wreck of the savings and loan industry almost put us out of business."

The pressure of Hank's high-risk business life was keeping him under constant stress. He knew he wasn't eating a healthy diet and that his genetic heritage put him at risk of a heart attack. Eventually his sense of responsibility to his family led Hank to take action to improve his health. It saved his life — but not in the way he might have expected.

"In December 1990 I was on a cholesterol control program that required me to have an entrance physical and two more at six-month intervals. Part of

By the time of the Great Depression of the 1930s, paralytic poliomyelitis was the most feared disease known. Polio struck fast, was incurable, and crippled its victims for life. Hobbling on crutches, rolling in wheelchairs, or lying immobile in giant iron lungs, the legions of sufferers grew, year after year. Even the exact mechanism of polio's transmission was a hotly debated subject for many years, so many areas were placed under strict quarantine when cases of the disease began to manifest themselves. Only the fear surrounding AIDS can rival the feelings people had about polio in the first half of this century.

Once the Sabin and Salk vaccines were proven effective in the '60s, the disease was quickly eradicated throughout most of the industrialized world. The economic effect has been enormous; it has been estimated that the polio vaccine pays for the cost of its development every three weeks. The benefit to the United States alone for this single breakthrough runs into the trillions of dollars. The social impact has been incalculable. The crutches, wheelchairs, and iron lungs of polio victims have at last been banished from children's and parents' nightmares, at least in the developed world.

Source: The Polio Information Center Online
(http://128.59.173.136/PICO/PICO.html)

the physical was a digital rectal exam, which indicated no problems with my prostate.

"At the end of 1991, after twelve months on the cholesterol reduction program, I made my annual January trip to Florida and ran into my former attorney, who was on radiation for prostate cancer. He was not having a very good time of it, so I made up my mind to get a PSA (prostate specific antigen) test when I got home. The results of that test, in the spring of '92, told me I had prostate cancer. And the biopsy confirmed it."

A NEW PROJECT

Hank was shaken by the diagnosis. But he had battled polio and come out on top, so he set out to learn all he could about this new disease and, with the support of his family, attack it head-on. He began to ask questions and gather information.

"The next thing that happened was really fortunate. While talking to another prostate cancer patient, I heard about US TOO!, the prostate cancer support group. It began with five guys who had started talking in doctors' waiting rooms at the University of Chicago Hospital about the

Men don't like to talk about prostate cancer. In general, if it's trouble below the belt, it's nobody's business. It's a threat to their masculinity, especially to those who grew up in the John Wayne/Mickey Spillane ethic of the '50s. Unwilling to admit vulnerability, they postpone physicals and avoid treatment — especially prostate treatment, which is understood to mean impotence.

But times change, and men change with them. Now there are places men can go, groups they can join, to discuss these fearful subjects with other men and get help making medical decisions. What are the consequences of this course of treatment, of that medicine? Nausea? Incontinence? Painful urination? "I know what the doc says, but what really happens?"

Rapid advances in medicine often turn the terrors of our grandfathers into mere campfire legends. Joining a support group can not only help men evaluate and accept sound medical advice — it can slay the dragons that kept men from seeking treatment and living out a long and healthy life.

side effects of treatment and other problems. Other hospitals heard about this, called US TOO!, and the second chapter was formed. Soon, other men at other hospitals asked US TOO! to come talk to them, and it wasn't long before we had grown to fifty chapters.

"I went to a meeting. I got my eyes and ears opened by hearing what others had gone through. As a result, I changed my ideas about what I wanted to do. I ended up getting a radical prostatectomy.

"But the more important thing was that I be-

Prostate gland: *a gland, found only in men, which produces some of the seminal fluid that protects and nourishes sperm cells. About the size of a walnut, it is located in front of the rectum, behind the base of the penis, and beneath the bladder.*

Prostate cancer: *a cancer that develops from cells of the prostate gland and may eventually spread to other parts of the body. Most prostate cancers grow very slowly. Autopsy studies show that many elderly men who died of other diseases also had a prostate cancer that neither they nor their doctors were aware of. But some prostate cancers can grow and spread quickly.*

Frequency of occurrence: *Prostate cancer is the most common cancer, excluding nonmelanoma skin cancers, in American men. US TOO! estimates that 190,000 new cases of prostate cancer will be diagnosed in the United States and that 32,000 men will die of it in the year 2000. Prostate cancer accounts for about 11 percent of cancer deaths in men, second only to lung cancer.*

Survivability: *Ninety-two percent of men diagnosed with prostate cancer survive at least five years, and 67 percent survive at least ten years. Fifty-eight percent of all prostate cancers are found while they are still localized (that is, confined to the prostate), and the five-year relative survival rate for men with localized prostate cancer is 100 percent. Thirty-one percent of prostate cancers have already spread locally (to tissues near the prostate) at the time of diagnosis. The five-year survival rate for these men is 94 percent. Among the 11 percent of men whose prostate cancers have already spread to distant parts of the body at the time of diagnosis, about 31 percent are expected to survive at least five years.*

came more involved in US TOO! I got interested in how men got together and talked, and I also felt I was giving back some of the benefit I got out of it. I went to the group meetings and participated, and I was invited onto the board. Then, when US TOO! was reorganized in 1993, I was elected chairman.

"The reason I was elected chairman was that the board wanted me to negotiate with some of the urologists in the East who had ideas about joining support groups. We didn't think that was a good

Digital rectal exam (DRE): an examination in which a doctor inserts a gloved, lubricated finger into the patient's rectum to feel for any irregular or abnormally firm area that might be a cancer. The prostate gland is located next to the rectum, and most cancers begin in the part of the gland that can be reached by a rectal exam. Though it may be uncomfortable, the exam causes no pain and takes only a short time. DRE is less effective than the PSA blood test in finding prostate cancer but can sometimes find tumors in men with normal PSA levels.

Prostate-specific antigen (PSA): a protein produced by prostate cells. The higher the PSA level, the more likely the presence of prostate cancer. PSA blood test results under 4 ng/ml (nanograms per milliliter) are usually considered normal, over 10 ng/ml high, and 4–10 ng/ml borderline. The American Cancer Society recommends that health care providers offer the PSA blood test and DRE yearly, beginning at age fifty, to men who have at least a ten-year life expectancy, and to younger men who are at high risk. Although the PSA test is not perfect, it is the best test currently available for early detection of prostate cancer. Since doctors started using this test, the number of prostate cancers found at an early, curable stage has increased.

Source: US TOO! (www.ustoo.org)

Today, there are many treatment options available, including prostatectomy, orchidectomy, cryotherapy, radiation therapy, hormone therapy, chemotherapy, and watchful waiting. The stage of the disease and lifestyle preferences affect treatment decisions, which should be made with your physician and family members.

idea. We thought support groups should be operated and controlled by patients.

"When I became chairman, we had no money. We hadn't had to raise any up to then because we had been supported indirectly by pharmaceutical companies. But those funds dried up, so we had to start doing our own fundraising. And that meant putting together a new organization. We did so. We got our first grant in 1994, and most of the companies that supported us at the beginning are still supporting us."

Part of the mission of US TOO!, Hank explains, is to provide international awareness, education, individual support, and political advocacy. "In 1993, we recruited men in other parts of the country as regional directors to help us set up and run chapters. Today we have about 500 chapters in twenty-five regions, and about 250,000 members, including wives and other family members. We have a monthly newsletter, the *Hot Sheet,* that is mailed to members and also gets copied and distributed to hospital waiting rooms and other places. And we have a monthly *Leader Letter* that gets mailed to chapter leaders and regional directors to tell them about upcoming programs, clinical trials, and so forth. We've also partnered with the National Cancer Institute to put out a packet of information, including a new booklet outlining what

The desire to "give back," to be engaged, to actively help others, is a common theme in this book and throughout the cancer community. Why? For one thing, the act of giving is just what your mother told you it was: more blessed than receiving.

For the patient, the gift of extended life, however long that may be, is seen as a second chance. Many take the opportunity to make a difference in the world — to lend a hand, offer encouragement, return a favor, make a phone call that should have been made years ago, or even to look a little longer at the sunset.

Hank will modestly tell you that he was encouraged to lead US TOO! because of his negotiating skills, but it was much more than that. It was his commitment to the interests of the members of this community, "our guys," that attracted others to his guidance.

prostate cancer is and what men can expect if they're diagnosed early, the various treatments, and the no-treatment option."

THE WAKE-UP CALL

"Often you'll hear men with prostate cancer saying things like, 'It's the best thing that ever happened to me,' or 'It woke me up.' Some of these things sound like exaggerations, but I think that when people are hit with cancer, they have considerable cause to reflect on how long they will be around, whether they've enjoyed life to the fullest, how they are going to use the time they have left, and so forth.

"Anyone who gets prostate cancer and stays alive for eight years, as I have, realizes that it's a gift and wants to go out and carry the word. And having had one previous experience with a disabling disease, I was probably better equipped to handle prostate cancer.

"On the other hand, there were times when I asked myself, Why did I come up with two whammies? I think the way you react is the

Radical prostatectomy: surgery to remove cancer from the prostate and from nearby areas to which it has spread. It is most often used during the cancer's early stages, when prostate cancer is located only within the prostate. Surgery may help prevent further spread of the cancer. If the cancer is small and located exclusively within the prostate, the surgery may cure the disease.

Advantages: Prostatectomy is a one-time procedure that may cure prostate cancer in its early stages and help extend life in the later stages.

Disadvantages: Prostatectomy is a major operation that requires hospitalization and can produce side effects, including impotence, incontinence (loss of urinary control), and narrowing of the urethra, which can make urination difficult. Impotence occurs in a high percentage of patients. In recent years, however, the percentage of men with impotence following surgery has decreased because of a new nerve-sparing surgical technique. Incontinence occurs in only a small percentage of patients.

Source: US TOO! (www.ustoo.com/options)

key to the rest of your life. If you're resentful, you affect your life negatively. If your reaction is to turn lemons into lemonade, that attitude tends to help your recovery."

AN OPEN-MINDED APPROACH

The mind-body connection is not something that men of Hank's generation readily embrace, but Hank sees its results every day. He believes men should pursue traditional medicine as well as promising alternatives in search of prevention, early detection, and treatment. "I take seriously the Surgeon General's study that showed how membership in a support group can actually make treatment more effective. Getting the support of others, and giving others support, completes some mind-body connection that makes whatever is being done work better.

"We've broadened the US TOO! mission statement to include advocacy. We think men should take a lesson from women, particularly in the area of breast cancer, and stump for more attention from the medical profession and the medical industry, and particularly from the federal government. Prostate cancer is the most frequently diagnosed male cancer, with the second highest mortality, and there's not enough money devoted to research. The only reason mortality is declining is because of the PSA, and because more men are being diagnosed early. So our first two missions are to make more people aware of prostate cancer and to push for more research into its treatment and cure.

"Our third mission is the real challenge: to reach men who have just been diagnosed with prostate cancer. It's really hard to get to them. We've tried appealing to doctors and urologists to tell their patients about our support group, but too often men don't hear about US TOO! until after they've been treated and are incontinent or impotent and very unhappy about it. If only we could get to these men and stress how important it is to communicate with the physician, they would not end up so unhappy when things don't turn out well. That's one of reasons we partnered with NCI — to provide more information to a larger population of men.

"Now, some men do better than others, and that's wonderful, because it's good for other men with prostate cancer to know. But a lot of the time, when men go through prostatectomy or radiation and think they're cured, their first impulse is to forget they ever had it and go on with living. Of course you don't want to go through life dwelling on the fact that you once had cancer, but we feel that if you've been lucky enough to come through it without problems, you owe it to other men to come talk about it and give them hope and advice — to serve as an example, and to strengthen the spirit of men who have not been so lucky.

"We deal with men who are undergoing treatment and recovering, and with some who get worse and eventually die. Helping these men through the difficult times right up to the end — it's tough, but it's a wonderful thing to be able to help. To see their appreciation is a reward that you don't get by just passing through life without caring for others.

"Whatever adversity hits you in life — and cancer is certainly one of the possibilities — you can feel pride if your reaction is to grab it by the neck and shake it and say to it, 'Not only are you not going to beat me, but you're not going to beat a lot of other people if I can help them.'"

Imagine this scenario: You find yourself, without warning, far out at sea in the aftermath of some terrible shipwreck, and you don't know how you got there. You are swimming, trying to stay afloat, amid piles of floating debris. All around you are men floating, cursing, weeping, fighting, swimming in circles, drowning.

What do you do? Do you let go of your rationality, give in to panic and self-pity, and join the circlers, the fighters, the drowners? No, you look around you for some way to survive. You see planks and ropes and pieces of twine. You pull yourself up on a shattered pallet and begin to pull together these shards of a lost vessel.

Before long, you've managed to construct a crude but seaworthy raft that you can control to an extent. You've even erected a primitive sail and find you can make headway toward the horizon.

This makes you an engineer.

Now: what do you do next? Do you look at the panic-stricken mob around you, shake your head, and set sail for the horizon? No, you stand up, speak in a firm voice, and get them to calm down. You instruct them to start gathering up more of the flotsam around them. You show them how to bind it together with bits of rope, how to make a crude but serviceable tiller, and how to rig a sheet so that each cobbled-together raft will go in the desired direction.

Then you speak to them in your most reassuring voice. You tell them there's land in that direction over there, somewhere beneath the tallest clouds, and that if everybody will stick together and watch out for each other, most of them will arrive and be rescued back into the land of the living.

This makes you a leader.

10

The Voice of a Father and Son

*In my dream, the angel shrugged & said, If we fail this time, it
will be a failure of imagination & then she placed the world
gently in the palm of my hand.*

Brian Andreas, *"Imagining World"*

APRIL 1962

I'M SITTING IN THE SCHOOL NURSE'S OFFICE at Tappan Junior High
School in Ann Arbor, Michigan. Why? Because I'm too worried to
remain in class — I need to talk with somebody. The nurse is kind;
she makes me feel safe. "It will be okay, Michael," she says.

My father, Orville Samuelson, is at the University of Michigan
Hospital having a cancerous lung removed. A heavy smoker all his
life, my dad, at fifty-three, is only beginning to suffer the consequences
of poor lifestyle choices. I'm fifteen and just beginning to follow his
example.

As a result of zillions of puffs on Winston cigarettes and a lifetime of alcohol abuse, my dad's next fifteen years are filled with
pain, frustration, a prescription drug–induced haze, and a zillion
more puffs on Winston cigarettes. Oh, he has bursts of creativity (he
is the original Mr. Fix-It) and fleeting moments of pleasure, but after
that spring day, the fire fades from his spirit as the energy drains
from his body.

Over the years, additional surgeries pull us back to the University of Michigan Hospital, including a series of horrific amputations
for peripheral artery disease. The years of smoking have broken down
the vessels needed to bring blood to his toes and feet. This eventually results in gangrene, leading to the removal of a toe, a foot, one

leg, and then the other leg. He stops drinking but keeps smoking. He has one more burst of energy and creativity: he rigs his old Buick Electra 225 to operate with hand controls. This illusion of independence is a dream that briefly puts the sparkle back in his eye. Unfortunately, he has time for only a couple of test runs before he dies at the University of Michigan Hospital at the age of sixty-seven. Invasive melanoma has been diagnosed in his stumps, and his heart can no longer take the assaults.

I remember him as a good man who loved his family, worked hard, and did his best. He certainly drank too much and smoked too much — but over that same fifteen years, so did I.

My father was not a philosophical man, nor, true to his Swedish heritage, did he show much affection or emotion. But shortly before he died, he beckoned me close to his bedside and spoke words I will never forget. He took my hand, looked at me with hollowed, steel-gray eyes, and said, with both sadness and parental urgency:

"In your hand you hold the most precious gift of all — the gift of life. You can nurture and grow it, or you can crumble it and throw it away. Either way, it's yours."

This was both advice and confession. I was thirty years old, and in all my life that was the only direct guidance I ever got from my dad. But it was powerful — and it took hold.

My dad might have been distracted during the crucial years of my development, but I got a great deal of support, love, and attention. I had a wonderful mother, Mary, who would remain a close friend until she died of emphysema at the age of eighty-three; my nine-years-older brother, Paul, to whom I looked up and for whom I cried for joy when he came home on his first leave from the Air Force; my kind and gentle sister Dodie, who was seven years older; and David, just two years older and forever a friend. I had a strong, protective foundation and many, many blessings.

"In your hand you hold the most precious gift of all — the gift of life. You can nurture and grow it, or you can crumble it and throw it away. Either way, it's yours."

Unfortunately, modeling a healthy lifestyle was not one of the blessings. Other smokers in the family included — well, everyone! This was the sixties and seventies, and everywhere you went you were encouraged to smoke. Arnold Palmer was dropping his L&M onto the green before making a long putt; major-league baseball players smoked in their dugouts; doctors told us that Camels helped our digestion; even Fred Flintstone and Barney Rubble would sneak off behind the garage for a Winston. My smoking was a foregone conclusion. However, within a year of my dad's death, that all changed.

REFORM

Reacting to forever-cold fingers and toes as well as the subconscious echo of my dad's parting gift, I quit smoking with the aid of Smoke Stoppers, a smoking cessation program. Within a few months, I left my job as a high-school guidance counselor with the Hartland, Michigan, school district and devoted all my professional energy to turning Smoke Stoppers into an international program (one that is now distributed to over 2 million people). Shortly after leaving the school system for the new field of health promotion, I must have heard my dad whispering to me one more time, because I decided that, given my family history and the fact that ice-cold beer was slowly moving from the shadows to the center of both my social and solitary activities, I turned my back on the Bud Man and walked away for good.

My colleagues and I then formed the National Center for Health Promotion and expanded our programs nationwide to include weight control, stress management, and exercise, along with smoking cessation. Eventually, we would train several thousands of health promotion instructors, who provided services throughout a network of hundreds of leading medical centers and corporations. In addition to administrative responsibilities, I spent the next twenty years traveling the country lecturing and writing on the importance of lifestyle management, medical self-responsibility, early detection, and early intervention.

Little did I know, when I was lecturing in Milwaukee, Miami, Boston, and Buffalo, that the message I was delivering, inspired by my father, would one day save my life.

APRIL 8, 1999

This one of those days you don't forget. I was getting ready to leave on a trip with my son Derek, but I had put off preparing my tax return, so I had to go to my accountant's office. And when I walked in and saw him, a man I had known for twenty-five years, he didn't look well. I said, "How are you feeling, Rod?" And Rod Byrne looked at me with a funny smile on his face and said, "Pretty good, pretty good." Then he said, "Uh . . . actually, I've been in chemotherapy."

That stopped me. I thought I must have heard him wrong, because that would mean he had cancer. I said, "What?" He said, "Yes, I had a radical mastectomy in February." And again I was hit with something I didn't think I had heard right, because when you hear "mastectomy," you immediately think of a woman.

I must have had quite a look on my face, because Rod said, "Yeah, it shocked the shit out of me, too!" And he laughed.

We sat down, and Rod told me his story. He had seen John Stossel talking about men's health on television. Remembering that I had mentioned working with Stossel when *20/20* featured Smoke Stoppers, and what a nice guy Stossel was, my accountant paid close attention. One of the things they talked about was a form of cancer that was rare in men — breast cancer.

The next day, in the shower, Rod Byrne, forty-three, remembered the TV show and checked himself. He found a lump. And it turned out to be stage-two invasive ductal carcinoma (there was no lymph node involvement, but the tumor was larger than 2 centimeters).

As I walked to my car, there on Main Street in Ann Arbor, Michigan, I did my very first breast self-exam.

I gave him a hug and said, "I'll say a prayer for you."

I left there thinking about Rod's unlikely cancer. As I walked to my car, there on Main Street in Ann Arbor, Michigan, I did my very first breast self-exam (you can do just about anything while walking down Main Street in Ann Arbor, Michigan), and I felt a hard lump behind my right nipple. It wasn't any bigger than a pea, but it was as hard as could be. There was no pain. Smiling at the power of suggestion, I got in my car and drove home. I told my wife about Rod, and I said, "Come here and feel this." She looked at me in a strange way, then she put her hand on my chest. She said, "Yeah, there's something there."

So the next day — because I had spent my professional life in health promotion talking about medical self-responsibility, early detection, and early intervention — I picked up the phone and called my primary doc, Bob Brakey, whom I've known for close to twenty years. He said, "Michael, don't worry about it, it's probably just a cyst. We can always squeeze you in, of course, so come on in."

I went in feeling embarrassed about calling attention to myself, no doubt needlessly, and taking up a professional's valuable time. But I felt compelled to go. As it turned out, he wasn't able to see me that morning, so I saw a colleague of his, a female physician, Toby Jacobowitz. I thought this was good, because as a woman she would have a more sensitive touch — at least that was my layperson thinking. She asked, "What are you here for, Michael?" I told her. She just shook her head and said, "In all my years of practice, I never ever have found a man with breast cancer. We studied a case back in medical school, but I've never run into one in my practice. I don't even screen for breast cancer in men much older than you."

This comforted me somewhat, but I still felt I wanted to get it checked out. She went ahead with a full breast exam, just as she would with a woman. She came to the area of the nipple and said, "Yeah, there's something there. It's probably just a cyst, but if you'd like peace of mind, here's a referral to a breast specialist."

I think 90 percent of guys at this point would have crumpled up that piece of paper and tossed it in the trash and thought, Boy, I'm glad I dodged that bullet, and then, having gone through the motions, just gone on with their lives. And that was my impulse, too. But all that time I had spent talking about health promotion and disease prevention compelled me to pick up the phone as soon as I got home.

I set up an appointment to come in right after my trip. Then my son and I went to England. Every once in a while I would think about it, about how unnecessary it was, but I would always come back to the fact that I had to find out.

When I got back, I went to see the surgeon, Dr. Manfred Marcus. I was sitting in his office, and it was all women, and again I felt I was taking up people's time. Then he came in and said, "Now, why are you here?" I explained it to him, and he said, "Your friend, he has breast cancer? So rare, so very rare," and shook his head.

During the exam, he said, "Yes, there's something there. It's probably just a sebaceous cyst. Nothing to worry about. What would you like to do?"

That shook me. I grew up in the fifties, when the doctor was god and you did what he said. And, in spite of my lectures on medical self-responsibility, a part of me wanted the answer to come from him. I said, "Excuse me?"

He said, "Well, we can do a mammogram, or we could just go ahead and take it out and do a biopsy."

I cringed at the memory of Hillary, my wife, telling me about the discomfort of her mammograms. Besides, I'm a guy — I thought I didn't have to do that kind of thing! So I said, "Take it out."

THE COLD TRUTH

A week later I went in for the biopsy. It was a beautiful day, and everybody was friendly and talking about upcoming Memorial Day barbecues and picnics. Besides Dr. Marcus, there were three people in the room with me saying, "Don't worry, it's probably just a cyst," and laughing and talking about softball and barbecue. It was a simple procedure, so I had a local anesthetic because I wanted to be awake.

Then they started the operation. And everybody stopped talking. All I could hear was the instruments clinking. The silence was deafening. It was surreal, a twilight-zone feeling. I was part of the scene — then I realized I *was* the scene. I knew there was something that nobody was talking about that was pretty scary. And I thought, Oh, shit.

They sewed me up. Then they had to reopen the incision because the bleeding wouldn't stop. They tried again, and still it wouldn't stop, so they had to cauterize the blood vessels. I found out later the bleeding was a bad sign. Tumors bleed like crazy; they're engorged with blood vessels, so the whole area bleeds heavily.

I didn't feel it, because I was numb, but I'll never forget the smell of that tissue being burned as if by a soldering iron. Everybody was gathered around, watching the procedure, nobody talking. Finally Dr. Marcus got the bleeding stopped and sewed me up. Then he put his hand on my shoulder and leaned over very close to my face, still with his mask on, and said, "Michael, I don't know what this is, but I don't think it's cancer."

Here was a highly regarded surgeon who did this several times a month, saying he didn't know what it was. That told me he *did* know what it was but needed to confirm it.

Unfortunately, this was Friday before Memorial Day weekend, which meant we would not get lab results until Tuesday. It was a very long weekend. When the day finally came, I was working around the house, and the phone rang. "Michael? This is Dr. Marcus." I knew from the tone of his voice I was not going to like what he had to say.

He said, "No good news. You have cancer." And then he said, "Worse news, you are at a high nuclear grade. You have a very aggressive cancer, and we have to see you immediately."

In the ten seconds between "Michael, no good news . . ." and "high nuclear grade," I reverted from fully alert back to my personal twilight zone. I remember saying, calmly, "Okay, fine. Uh, what does that mean? What's our next step?" I was being very clinical, very analytical, very male. He said, "I need you to come in tomorrow morning." I said, casually, "You name the time, I'll be there." He said, "Be here at ten."

So my work with John Stossel had come full circle. If I had not worked with John, I would not have mentioned it to the accountant, and he wouldn't have stopped what he was doing and paid attention to the television show, and he wouldn't have found his cancer and mentioned it to me and caused me to find my cancer.

HIDING FROM IT

I hung up the phone. I was alone in the house, surrounded by absolute stillness and silence. The thought came to me that my children would be home soon. I couldn't face them right away — they would be full of energy and enthusiasm as usual, and I knew I couldn't handle that. So I put on my running shoes and went out for a run. I got maybe fifty yards, and all the energy drained out of my body and I slowed to a walk. Then I tried to run again but couldn't do anything more than walk, and when I turned the corner I saw Hillary's car coming, and it was the most beautiful sight I could remember ever seeing.

At that moment I needed nothing more than to see her. She stopped the car and gave me a big smile and I got in. I couldn't look at her at first, but then I turned to her and said, "I've got cancer." Then I started to cry.

What got to me was not the thought of dying — it was the idea of not seeing my children grow up, not seeing my friends, not being a part of the future. And being with Hillary let me express those fears.

And she was wonderful. She didn't cry, but she comforted me, which was exactly what I needed. And she said, "We're going to beat this."

NEW PRIORITIES

When I went in to see the doctor the next morning, I was back in my practical, analytical frame of mind. I said, "Okay, what do we have to do?" He said, "Well, in your case there's only one option. We have to do a radical mastectomy."

Keep in mind that four weeks before this I had barely heard of breast cancer in men, and here I was facing radical surgery. I said, "Well, let's see, I've got a speech in New Jersey, I've got one in Kansas City, so . . . let's schedule this for the end of June." And the doctor said, "Michael, you don't have until the end of June. It's very aggressive. It's growing very, very fast. It can go to the lungs, the liver, or the brain, and it may already have done that. You don't have thirty days to do this. We need to schedule it immediately."

I said, "Let's compromise, then. Let me do one speech, and we'll schedule the surgery in two weeks." He shook his head: "I don't recommend that." And I said, "We're going to do this, but let's do it this way."

I went home, and I thought about it, and I talked with my wife, who told me I was crazy. I called one of my associates, told him the situation, and said, "I've got to give one speech but I need to find someone else to do the others. Will you help me out?" He said, "Michael, that's stupid. You're not giving any speeches. You're going to call the doctor back and have the surgery." I said, "No, it's okay, I've got a couple of weeks."

And he said, "Michael, if somebody had just said to you that your wife or one of your children had just been diagnosed with cancer and needed surgery as soon as possible, would you say let's postpone it for a couple of weeks while I go give a speech?"

My associate was right. The decision to postpone was stupid. I said, "Thank you," and hung up the phone. Then I called Dr. Marcus's office and said, "As soon as you have an opening and can schedule an operating room, let's do it." We scheduled my surgery for June 14th.

I did one more important thing before agreeing to the surgery. Dr. Marcus seemed very professional, and he was certainly courteous, but I knew very little about his skill or reputation. I called my primary physician and asked him who he would recommend for the surgery. He said, "Michael, all I can tell you is that when my mother-in-law needed a mastectomy, I sent her to Manfred Marcus." That was all I needed to hear.

TELLING ALL

The Saturday before surgery was my son's high-school graduation party, and I didn't want to tell the children until after that. But a friend said, "They have a right to know. Besides, they'll know anyway, and their imagination will make it worse than it is. You owe it to them to tell them."

So we sat down with the children before the graduation party and told them what was going on. We have a very loving household with open communication. We talked about what it meant, and that we were catching it while it was still small, and that I would have to have a mastectomy and would be sick for a while but there was a strong probability that I would recover completely. My sixteen-year-old daughter, Logan, kind of laughed and said, "You know, only my dad would end up with one boob." Everybody gave me a hug, and Derek, seventeen, came up and said, "Dad, this is a no-brainer. You're going to be fine." And never for a second did he think anything else. The next day, however, my daughter broke down in school and had to come home.

We called my oldest son, Brent, twenty-three at the time, who lives in Kalamazoo, Michigan. He drove home and with beautiful hesitation let me know that if I had chemotherapy and needed any marijuana for the nausea, he could get it for me. I smiled, we hugged, and I told him that I loved him and appreciated the offer. I have learned over the years that there are times for fatherly lectures and there are times for hugs. This was a time for a hug.

For friends and family out of town, the hugs were virtual but no less meaningful. Letters, cards, flowers, books, and prayers came from as far away as Korea and Sweden. Colleagues Larry Chapman, David Hunnicutt, and Elaine Sullivan offered prayers and volunteered to fill my speaking commitments. Michael O'Donnell made it very clear that I would not quietly accept whatever was to come but that I would, instead, actively fight the cancer with my mind, body, and spirit. My brothers and their families kept a constant long-distance vigil, and their prayers and thoughts were always a comfort. And once, when I saw myself inching a little closer toward the edge, I felt my mother's arms reaching out to hold me. I knew then that I would be fine.

I had the surgery, then continued to have wonderful support from everybody — family, friends, and colleagues — during my recovery. A dear friend and business colleague of mine over the last twenty

Although the disease is rare in men, about one percent of all breast cancers do occur in men. Approximately 1,300 new cases of male breast cancer were diagnosed in 1999, and there were about 400 deaths. Breast cancer in males is evaluated, staged, and treated exactly as it is for women. The pathology, prognostic indicators, and overall survival rates are similar to female breast cancer as well.

years had T-shirts made that said, "Fuck Cancer." It was cryptic, so as not to be overtly offensive, but it was there if you looked closely. And it was perfect. It expressed not only humor, which is very important when you're dealing with cancer, but also defiance — the attitude that the cancer was not going to win this fight. And it was a wonderful icebreaker to encourage people to talk about it.

As I was being wheeled into surgery, I knew that I would live, and I told everybody around me that someday I would write a book about the experience. It was too important a story to keep hidden.

In the eighteen months since then, I've spent my time finding opportunities to be a voice for other citizens of our town — the cancer community — and an advocate for medical self-responsibility, early detection, and early intervention. I've co-hosted a number of Internet cancer talk shows for the American Cancer Society, served as the chairman of the National Consumer Advisory Council for cancerfacts.com, been part of the National Dialogue on Cancer that was formed by President and Barbara Bush, and been involved with the Internet Health Care Coalition, an organization dedicated to providing accurate, timely information to patients and caregivers. It's been a blessing to be a part of this process.

I've learned something else, too. Decisions have never been clearer in my life. The ambiguity is gone. We all have a sense of what is right, what is important, what's dangerous, what's enriching, what's threatening — but coming face-to-face with death lets you tune in to it. It's like going from being myopic to having 360-degree peripheral vision with surround sound. You pick up things earlier on your radar screen. And you don't suppress your visceral response any more. Instead of overanalyzing, you go with your gut when it tells you what's right and what's wrong.

A HAND ON MY SOUL

When I was going through this, I had incredible love and support from family and friends, but the most powerful single moment happened with a total stranger, and it took me back to the safe harbor I found in Tappan Junior High School on that April afternoon in 1962.

A few weeks after the surgery, I was having a follow-up visit with Dr. Brakey. Before the doctor came in, a nurse was taking my temperature and blood pressure. I had never met her before, and my guess was that she was in her early sixties. She asked me how I was doing — and I told her.

In addition to pain from severe "cording" (shrinking of dried lymph vessels in my arm resulting from the node dissection) and the discomfort of having had the drainage tube removed from my chest, I was feeling depressed and exhausted. The impact of the past several weeks was creating a large black hole, and I could feel the suction building. Just as on that day nearly forty years ago, I needed to talk to somebody and, once again, here was a nurse willing to listen. She listened to my calm voice, but she also heard the silent cries within me. As she sat there in her traditional nurse's white uniform, she focused on me and only me. When I finished, she came over and put her hand on top of my hand and gave it a little squeeze. She looked at me and said, "You're going to be fine." That was all — a touch, eyes filled with compassion, and just the right words. It meant everything to me.

When she touched me, the transfer of energy and was palpable. It was as if this white-haired guy in his fifties had suddenly been replaced by this eight-year-old boy who had been hiding inside me, scared to death at what was going on, and who suddenly felt it was safe to come out of hiding. Every hair on my body stood on end.

She started to leave the room, then came back and kissed me on the cheek. Me and the eight-year-old boy. Then she said, "I probably shouldn't have done that, should I?" I said, "Thank you. It was wonderful."

And I thought: Science may have saved my life, but she just lifted my spirit. She touched my soul.

UPPERS

As have so many others in our community, I have learned that humor is great medicine. The situations I have found myself in, although deadly serious in their implications, have often seemed more than faintly ridiculous to me, as well as to others.

After my surgery, I had to go in for a mammogram of my remaining breast. I walked into this lovely pink room filled with women. They were all looking at me, and I was enjoying it, because their looks were saying, "What are you doing here?" I wasn't embarrassed, but I was clearly a sore thumb in that room, and it struck me as funny.

The nurse came out with a chart, looked around the room several times, and said, "Michelle Samuelson?" And this six-foot-two, 200-pound "Michelle" stands up and says, "I think you mean 'Michael,' and that would be me." She looked at me with a combination of embarrassment and pity, and said, "Oh, I'm sorry, sir." And I smiled and said, "Well, me too."

She led me to the mammogram machine, and I had to squat down to get into position for the machine to do its work. I've heard women talk about how uncomfortable the process is, and I don't have a lot of breast tissue, but the technician got what there was and squeezed and squeezed and I said, "I think you've probably squeezed enough." And she said, "Oh no, sir, we can go a little more." And she did.

An oncologist friend of mine sent me a cartoon that shows a man in a hospital gown standing in front of a machine that has obvious similarities to — and one obvious difference from — a mammogram machine. When Hillary first saw the cartoon, she laughed and said, "Touché!"

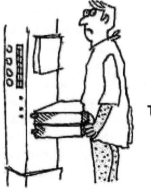

IF WOMEN CONTROLLED MEDICINE

The Manogram

As a man with a predominantly female disease, I am having an interesting experience getting in touch with my feminine side — perhaps more than I would have chosen. I am on Tamoxifen, a drug that was tested in clinical trials on 30,000 women but no men and is known to suppress the spread of breast cancer. One of the side effects is that it mimics menopause. It didn't take long for me to realize that I was putting the "men" into menopause, because I had the same reactions that a woman would have: night sweats, hot flashes, mood swings. My wife thinks this is wonderful. After all, how many couples get to share menopause? When we go somewhere, she will turn to me and say, "Is it warm in here?" and I'll look at her like she's crazy and say, "Who are you asking? Fifteen minutes ago it was, but now I'm freezing in my sweat." And we laugh. She thinks every man should go on Tamoxifen for at least six months just to see what menopause is all about.

THE CONDUIT

Sometimes I feel I am on a prepackaged collective journey, and that the experiences of many others are all going through me — that, in a way, I've been tapped to be a voice for others in our town. And there's not a shred of arrogance in this — in fact, it's rather frightening at times. It's a responsibility I take seriously. It's as if everything I've done in my life has led up to my being able to provide this voice.

Responsibility is an interesting word. It really means that you need to think of things other than yourself — things like family, friends, and community. It means that you need to believe in a universe where more than ME exists. I understand the notion that everything begins with ME; however, if you get too egocentric, you lose perspective on what is truly important. Yes, you need to feel good and contented, but I believe, more and more, that this contentment comes easier and is deeper when you help others. We need to celebrate the fact that helping others feels good! Altruism is neither exploitation nor self-sacrifice; it is the natural order of things. After all, if we are all one and connected, is it not in our best interest to help each other? It is selfishness, in the very best sense of the word.

Wherever I go in this world, I hear other voices sending me life lessons from the edge. They are reflective voices, filled with wisdom, pain, joy, confusion, appreciation, and acceptance. Sometimes these voices are whispers or shy giggles, sometimes shouts or angry cries or sardonic laughter. There are thousands of these voices, anxious to share, to teach. All we have to do is listen and pay attention.

My father was fifty-three when he was diagnosed with cancer and began a fifteen-year downward spiral ending in death. This coming spring, I will turn fifty-three. I don't know what future years will hold, but I'm starting them with a trip to Alaska with my son Derek. We plan to trek through glacier fields and climb a mountain. And when we get to the top of that mountain, I will take that last step on behalf of all the members of my cancer community, and I will say a prayer of gratitude for the gifts they have given me and for simply being alive. I will then look for new peaks, ponder the possibilities — and whisper to my father: "Thanks, Dad. You taught me more than you or I ever realized."

Epilogue: Journey to Another Edge

SOUTH DAVIDSON GLACIER
ALASKA
UNITED STATES OF AMERICA
CONTINENT OF NORTH AMERICA
WESTERN HEMISPHERE
EARTH
SOLAR SYSTEM
UNIVERSE
THE MIND OF GOD

AUGUST 13, 2000

6:30 A.M.

The cold damp stillness is broken by a rhythmic crunching and padding sound coming from just inches above my head. In that foggy place where you try to capture the fleeting echoes of sleep, the sound is both comforting and confusing. Dig-scoop-pour-pad, dig-scoop-pour-pad, dig-scoop-pour-pad, dig-scoop-pour-pad. What the . . . ?

Then I remember what Darsie told us yesterday when we set up camp: "Keep the tent posts covered in fresh snow so they won't come loose and pull out." A Good Samaritan with a shovel is the answer to my early morning question.

Darsie, Bill, and Chris are guides, from the Haines-based Alaska Mountain Guides and Climbing School, into whose hands my son, Derek, and I will entrust our health and safety for the next four days. Seven other mountaineers-in-training, ranging in age from early twenties to mid-fifties, will do the same.

Darsie, an environmental science graduate from Western Washington University, looks more like an accountant than a guide with fifteen years of mountain experience. He is the cofounder of the school and is clearly competent and in control. Bill studied zoology at the University of Washington and conveys an equal sense of confidence and knowledge. Chris is a rugged ten-year veteran of the marines who dropped out of flight school and left the military service when he realized that training to kill was not how he wished to move forward in life. All three are friendly, positive guys in their late twenties and early thirties.

"Hot drinks in ten minutes!" yells Bill from the kitchen, a spot we hollowed out of the snow when we first arrived on the south end of the Davidson Glacier. This is the signal to throw on our boots, gaiters, extra layers of fleece, Gore-Tex jackets, pants, hats, and gloves. Then we unzip the flaps to the vestibule and the outer opening of our two-man tent and walk out onto the prehistoric block of ice and snow.

And so our summer day begins.

Before we get to our hot chocolate, we pass four other tents that look just like ours: multicolored bumps on a pure white background. The first tent houses James, an art dealer and Good Samaritan from North Carolina; Richard, a computer consultant from Australia; and Duane, a dairy farmer and sled-dog breeder from Wisconsin. The next tent is shared by Avi, a computer consultant from South Africa; Derek, a riverboat pilot from Juneau; and Mosby, an English teacher heading to an American school in Switzerland. Next is Penn's tent; Penn is a physician from the United Kingdom and our group's only female mountaineer. The guides' tent, a snow lounge, and the kitchen make up the remaining structures in our little community. Of course, we also have a snow latrine complete with a privacy wall, and a distant "pee wand" that reminds us to limit our areas of contamination.

After a quick breakfast of cold cereal and hot English muffins, we return to our tents, pick up our ice axes, drink more water (hydration is critical in the mountains), smear on plenty of sunscreen and lip protection, and put on our protective helmets. Then, formed up into three four-person rope teams, we head for the slope behind us to practice self-arrest techniques. These exercises consist of learning what to do in case you lose your balance and begin to fall down an icy mountain. For about two hours we practice falling on our backs, bellies, and butts as we learn to stop the fall by jabbing our axes into the slope. The guides make the time enjoyable as well as instructive, but this is clearly serious business. Failure to instinctively stab the ice after a sudden fall could result in serious injury or death.

The time on the slope is interesting, fun (especially watching my man-child sliding down the hill — not unlike when he was a little boy), and also fatiguing. Since the cancer diagnosis, surgery, and the beginning of hormone therapy, I have long periods of strength and stamina but also daily bouts of body-slamming exhaustion. A quick timeout of twenty minutes or so is all I usually need to bounce back, but I can't always predict when the irresistible urge to lie down will hit me. Sometimes I forget that I am still a cancer patient. Later that afternoon, I will be reminded.

11:30 A.M.

A quick lunch of chicken soup and peanut-butter-and-jelly sand-wiches is followed by more hot drinks and a lecture on crevasse res-cue techniques. The Davidson Glacier is criss-crossed with fissures from a few inches to several feet wide — and deeper than most of us care to contemplate. In some, the echo of a falling object never reaches the surface. Our guides are experienced and know what to look for, but that in no way guarantees that we will not fall or be pulled into an abyss. We pay close attention.

Once formed into our rope teams, we head out toward what can only be described as the single most beautiful view I have ever seen. The mountains towering above, the heavenly cloudscape below, and the pure white virginal canvas stretched before us set a majestic yet surreal scene that cannot be described — only experienced. Add in fresh, sweet air that you can taste, and congenial companions, and the stage is set for an extraordinary day.

We walk single file out of camp and head for the long pristine valley and the beckoning white slopes that gradually expose the jagged black peaks of the Fairweather Range. Standing guard is the regal

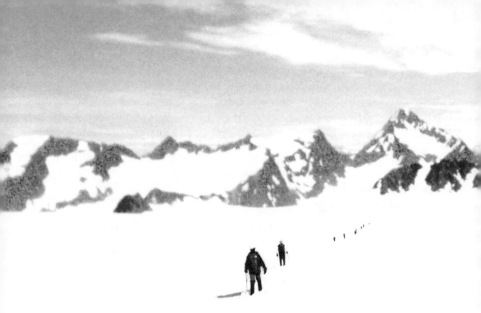

silhouette of Mount Fairweather, rising 15,300 feet into the deep, deep blue Alaskan sky.

For the next two hours only the sounds of boots breaking snow, hopelessly inadequate cameras clicking, and childlike expressions of awe break the silence of the glacier. The view constantly changes; the wind whips snow and clouds, and the sun dances with shadows. I can't decide which is more beautiful, the view around me or the reflection of that view in my son's eyes. On second thought, yes, I can.

As we approach our first peak, the slope gets progressively steeper and we have to zigzag upward. Physically, this requires that I shift my focus from the scene around me to the footprint trail in front of me. In spite of my months of training and a lean diet that has trimmed me by more than thirty pounds, the buoyancy fueled by adrenaline, inspiration, and beauty is giving way to muscle fatigue and that all-too-familiar urge to simply lie down and rest. At home, this would mean moving twenty yards from my study to the bedroom. But I am not on Village Road in Saline, Michigan — I am on the Davidson Glacier in Southeast Alaska. Rest, at this moment, is not an option — at least not to the primordial ancestor that pushes (harasses) me to continue and not complain.

Fortunately, my cardiovascular system is strong enough to deal with the altitude and exertion. The lungs that I abused with tobacco from age fifteen to thirty have recovered significantly over the past

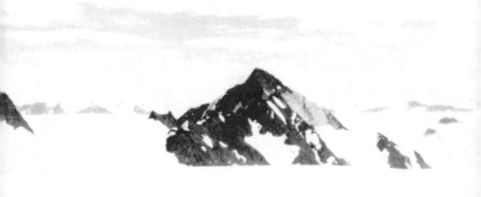

twenty-two smoke-free years. Years of studying meditation and deep-breathing techniques enable me to shift my focus from the growing muscle pain and fatigue to the task at hand: slogging, step by slow, painful step, closer and closer to the top. I watch the rope that connects me to Penn, and as it moves, so do I. For several minutes, the universe is reduced to the snakelike crawling of a 10-millimeter rope.

Then the snake stops. I look up; the team ahead of us has reached the peak. I take a deep breath, wipe the sweat off my face, and smile. I've made it!

With renewed strength, I unclip my harness from the team rope and begin the small rock-climb to the top ledge. The rock is very loose; it crumbles beneath my feet. Now is not the time for carelessness. I slow down, find my footing, and climb to meet Derek, who has already sprinted to the top as nimbly as a mountain goat. As I take that last step, I remember my pledge to honor those cancer survivors who have inspired me to take this trip, and I say a short prayer of thanks. And, oh yes, my dad and I have a wonderful chat. . . . The tears are cold as the wind strikes my face, but my smile and heart are oh, so warm.

4:15 P.M.

After a nice long rest, lots of water, and more sunscreen, we are ready to move on to another peak. I am now confident that I have

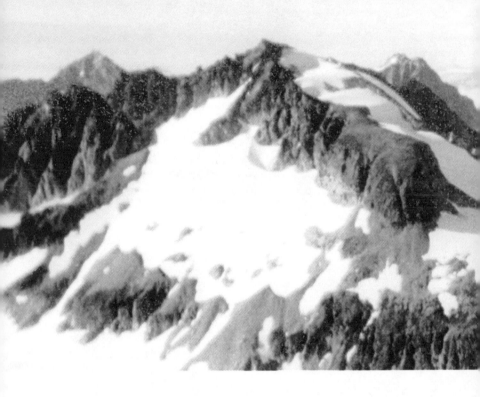

the strength to go all day. I am also a fool in need of advanced lessons in humility and the virtue of accepting the help of others. I will soon receive both lessons.

The others in my rope party are fine, but for me the way down the slope is more like a controlled fall then a smooth descent. The idea is to lead with the heel of your boot as you build a downward rhythm. To help stabilize each step, it's often easier to break new snow than to follow in someone else's tracks. Of course you are also keenly aware that the beaten path has passed the "no crevasse here" test and that breaking fresh trail runs a certain risk. I need to preserve as much strength as possible, so I accept the small risk and make my own bootprints.

There are two teams in front of ours, and I am the third member on our rope, so I can see all but one member of the entire group. Their descent is smooth and measured. They appear to be gliding effortlessly down to the valley. I, on the other hand, am running down the slope to keep the rope between me and Penn from becoming a clothesline. There is no grace in my step, no rhythm. This is work, and my quadriceps burn with each clumsy plunge. When we reach

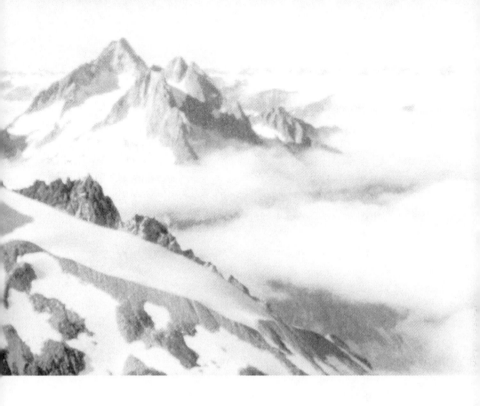

the bottom and begin our flat traverse of the valley, Penn hollers
back, "Are you all right, love?" I smile and lie as I tap my helmet to
signal that all is well.

More water, more sunscreen, more pictures. We trek across the
valley floor toward the next peak. Hey, I'm fine! No need for rest. No
need to ask Chris, our rope guide, to slow down the pace. I can keep
up with anybody. Look at me, I'm a mountaineer!

Then, after about an hour, we begin the second ascent of the
afternoon.

I make the mistake of focusing on how steeply we must climb to
get to the top. For an experienced mountaineer this is a small in-
cline, but what I see is Mount Everest. I stop seeing the beauty of the
glacier; I fixate on every step and the the way the rope is moving.
Several times I feel my legs starting to buckle — they are screaming
for a rest — but instead of listening to my body, I respond by increas-
ing my spot-focus meditation and denying my pain. Again and again,
Penn feels the tug of fatigue on the rope and hollers back, "Are you
all right, love? Do you need to rest?" And each time, the idiot inside
me reaches up and taps my helmet. I refuse to hold the team up; to

call attention to myself; to admit that I need help. I think of all the cancer survivors and the pain that so many of them have to endure. In comparison, this is just a single gnat in Paradise. I hear the words that are drilled into the head of every boy raised in the 1950s: "No pain, no gain." "Tough it out." "Quit your complaining." "Don't be a sissy." And, of course, I remember the words of Sister Mary Ada, who told us to offer our suffering up to the poor souls in Purgatory. I smile at the thought and figure that I must be flooding the gates of Heaven with newly purified souls, ready for entry.

When the snake pauses for more than a few seconds, I realize that the first team has reached the summit and that soon I will be able to rest. When it's my turn to "come on up!" I take off my harness and collapse in the snow. The others continue the short rock-climb to the view of the other side, but I do not move; cannot move; will not move. I hear their excitement at the vista spread out before them; I hear them urging me to come see. But I don't care. I do not move; cannot move; will not move. Beauty is for later. Now, I need to rest, lick my wounds, and feel sorry for myself. I will be fine. But for now — I do not move; cannot move; will not move.

Chris is concerned. He stays behind to talk with me. We talk about the cancer treatment; how great it is that I get to do this with one of my sons; his time in the military; the challenges of the mountain. We also talk (or, rather, he talks and I listen) about the importance of letting him know exactly how I am doing. We can slow down and take breaks whenever I need. The important thing is that I let him know. I can handle the physical challenge, he says, as long as I am honest about how I am feeling. Chris is compassionate without being patronizing, and it is greatly appreciated. So is the break. I am now ready to climb the last few yards and see what's on the other side.

As I reach the top and look out over the tops of clouds toward the Cathedral Peaks, my pain and fatigue melt away. Visibility is infinite and the view is like nothing I have ever seen before. I'm standing on the edge of the world, feeling awe, wonder, gratitude, and, most of all, an indescribable spiritual awareness. What a gift this is! I must treasure and respect the offering. I know, too, that this gift is not mine alone. I am accepting it on behalf of all who would be here if they could. Without their energy and inspiration I would not have made this trip; I would not have climbed this mountain peak; I would not have gained this moment.

Darsie is telling us to put on our harnesses and packs; it is time to climb down and return to base camp. I do not move; cannot move; will not move. But of course I must — and, with hesitation, I do.

7:45 P.M.

This descent is no more graceful than the last, but there is a difference. When we reach the floor of the valley, Penn needs to stop to remove a layer of fleece. Chris asks me if the pace is okay or should he slow it down. I begin to raise my hand to pat my helmet, but I stop halfway and say: "Please slow it down just a bit." I am learning.

Assuming ideal conditions, the journey back to camp will take about two hours. After about an hour, intense fatigue sets in once more and my steps are mixed with stumbles. It is a slow march across the floor of the glacier, the crunch of the snow serving as a metronome. At one point I look up and see that we are about to descend into a cloud. In this inexperienced mountain climber from the lower forty-eight, it triggers only appreciation of the spectacular view. To a guide, it means something else — the prospect of a total white-out, a combination of sun, mist, and snow that all but obliterates visibility. In the late afternoon on a glacier with dangerous crevasses and a

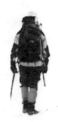
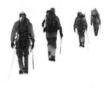

tired team of new climbers, this is a serious situation. We will need the keenest instincts and skills of our guides to avoid getting lost and stranded.

Penn, who is only forty feet in front of me, begins to fade into the mist. Chris has already disappeared. The scene is dreamlike, surreal, and — in my happy ignorance — simply wonderful. At one point the sun is a perfect circle of light piercing the thick mist. The result is the opposite of a shadow: instead of shade in a field of sunshine, there is a small pool of light shining on the snow, like a flashlight piercing the night. I feel the way I did when I was a child in church. I can sense a presence that is both comforting and frightening — not in a scary way, but in the knowledge of its awesome power and force. I have never felt more vulnerable; strangely, neither have I ever felt more safe.

The irony of my sense of security soon becomes apparent. We reach the next crest to find the other two rope teams formed in a circle. The white-out has made further travel impossible. We are amid crevasses, and we are lost.

I quickly find Derek, who is a little tired, like everyone else, but okay. The three guides huddle; the rest of us stand and speculate. There is a real possibility that we will have to tighten the circle and wait until the storm has cleared, even if it takes all night.

Still, I feel safe. I have not a clue which way to go, but it seems everyone else does. Fortunately, one of these is Chris. His training as a guide and his experience as a marine help him locate our outbound tracks. Soon, we are lined up in single file heading, once again, into the mist. Duane from Wisconsin feels we are going away from camp, but my money is on Chris.

10:00 P.M.

After a long fifteen minutes, I hear relieved voices and see the beginnings of shadows of small bumps on a pure white background. We're back! By the time we reach camp and collapse in the snow beside our tents, I hear the glorious sound of Bill's voice shouting, "Hot drinks in ten minutes!" Then I hear my own voice saying: "Thanks, God, it's been quite a summer's day."

AUGUST 20, 2000

As I sit in my comfortable study back in Michigan, I think about the days on the glacier and the number of times I used the lessons taught me by the voices in this book:

Determination. Perhaps most striking is Tim's voice. When you first look at the first peak we climbed, it seems impossible that anyone could get to the top. About 100 yards below the summit is very wide crevasse. To try to climb this peak head-on would be suicide. However, out of sight there is another route to the top. It takes longer and the path is difficult and tiring, but with determination you can reach the top — and the reward is spectacular. Tim knows this.

Humor. Without humor, stay home! A trip to the pee wand in the middle of the night with horizontal freezing rain has to make you smile, even if retrospectively. I can hear Lillie laughing already.

Discovery. When we turned into the valley and I looked up at the deepest blue sky I have ever seen, the first person that came into my mind was Lou — and I held my glance just a little longer than usual. This sky is for you, Lou.

Empowerment. Fern's philosophy of listening to your own voice made this trip possible. Years ago, I had a foot injury from too much (or improper) running. The physician I first saw told me to get comfortable shoes and forget about strenuous exercise. He said I had broken the "bubble warp" in my heel and it would never support my full weight. He was wrong. It was an injury that, with time and good foot support, I would recover from and be able to resume an active lifestyle. I found this out by listening to my own voice and getting a third opinion — mine being the first. I sent photos of myself on the glacier to both physicians, with messages of both thanks and polite caution.

Engagement. Matthew's advice to be part of your world, to jump in with both feet, to be a player, not just an observer, was exemplified by everyone on the glacier. Yes, there are risks in climbing mountains (of any kind), but when appropriate precautions are taken, the rewards are immeasurable.

Wisdom. There is the knowledge that comes from books and the wisdom that comes from experience. Reading about hypothermia,

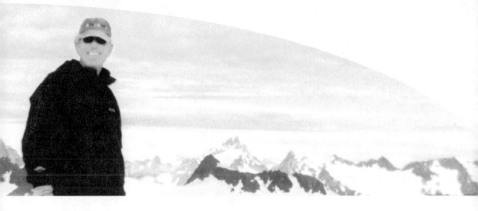

bush plane rides, glaciers, solitude, relationship building, and survival are not the same as living through sixty hours of freezing rain in a two-man tent; touching mountain peaks with a pilot who loves his plane more than anything in this world; a single night on the Davidson Glacier; five days without the sound of television, traffic, sirens, or even the morning music of a bird; living with strangers on an ice field; or wandering tied to a rope in a white-out. Ricky knows this.

Resilience. Doug taught me all I need to know about resilience.

Spirit. I was able to plan and complete this trip due in large part to my belief that I could do it. Yes, it was challenging, and there were moments when I would have preferred not to continue, but they were just moments. If I had let the negative thoughts and the pain take control, I would never had made it past the training phase. As Paula knows, a strong spirit and a few informal chats with God will take you a long, long way.

Leadership. Without competent and trustworthy leadership, we would have perished on the glacier. As Hank did for "his guys," Darsie, Bill, and Chris gave us the tools needed to survive. And we had the strength of comradeship: I could not look at the rope teams or our linked tents and not be reminded of cancer support groups like US TOO! We were all independent on the slope — and, at the same time, critically connected with real lifelines.

Father and Son. No words to describe this one. Derek and I were a couple of buddies on a glacier, but more — a father and his son, surrounded by the love and spirit of his brother Brent, his sister Logan, and his mother Hillary. We were quite a crowd up there.

Next stop — Nepal!

Michael Hayes Samuelson is the president of Samuelson & Associates, a management consulting firm that specializes in personal and professional productivity. Before this, Michael directed the National Center for Health Promotion (NCHP), an organization he cofounded in 1977. Over the years, NCHP earned a reputation as an international leader in the design and delivery of health management programs and instructor materials. As president and CEO, Michael led his marketing team to provide services to over 1,000 corporations and 800 medical centers, and directed a program of development and training for over 4,500 health promotion instructors in the United States, Canada, and Japan. He is a director and advisor to numerous prestigious boards and health organizations, including the Wellness Councils of America, Healthy Competition, HealthLift, Focus Health, and Nexcura. A well-respected and popular keynote speaker, Michael is viewed as a leader in health development, maintenance, and responsibility. He is a frequent guest lecturer at the University of Michigan and has developed and contributed to corporate health promotion policies for major U.S. corporations. A graduate of the University of Michigan with a master of arts degree in education, Michael is widely published and has appeared on over 200 television and radio stations throughout North America and has been interviewed by numerous print publications, including *Newsweek*, *USA Today*, and the *Wall Street Journal*. His work in the area of behavior change and health care consumer advocacy has been featured on the ABC News program *20/20*, the *Early Show* on CBS, and on CNN and MSNBC. In addition, Michael is a frequent guest host for the American Cancer Society's Cancer Survivor Network; a contributing author of the internatonal eHealth Code of Ethics; and, at the request of former President George Bush and Mrs. Bush, a collaborating partner with the National Dialogue on Cancer. To inquire about Michael's speeches and seminars, please call 734-429-3065.

Samuelson & Associates is a management consulting firm specializing in the design and delivery of presentations, trainings, and retreats focused on personal and professional productivity.

Presentations: Customized multimedia presentations that are motivating, inspirational, and informative. Topic areas included:

- Leadership
- High Performance Balance
- Wellness
- Adversity as an Asset
- Personal and Organizational Change
- Living, Working, and Playing with the Person Behind the Disease

Trainings: Half-day to two-day trainings in any of the above areas.

Retreats: Customized escape weekends where the focus is on balance and productivity.

For more information call 734-747-9579.